ADVANCED STRATEGY
FOR MEDICAL PRACTICE LEADERS

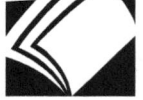

FINANCIAL
MANAGEMENT
EDITION

TAYA GORDON
MBA, FACMPE, CMOM

KEM TOLLIVER
FACMPE, CPC, CMOM

MGMA
104 INVERNESS TERRACE EAST
ENGLEWOOD, CO 80112-5306
877.275.6462
MGMA.COM

Inspiring
healthcare
excellence.℠

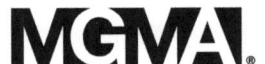

MGMA®

Published by: Medical Group Management Association (MGMA)

Library of Congress Control Number: 2022905955

Item: 1048
ISBN: 978-1-56829-036-2

Printed in the United States of America

10 9 8 7 6 5 4 3 2 1

Advanced Strategy for Medical Practice Leaders

Volume 1: Financial Management Edition

Volume 2: Human Resources Management Edition

Volume 3: Operations Management Edition

Contents

Acknowledgements

Taya Gordon

"The greater danger for most of us lies not in setting our aim too high and falling short; but in setting our aim too low, and achieving our mark."

—*Michelangelo*

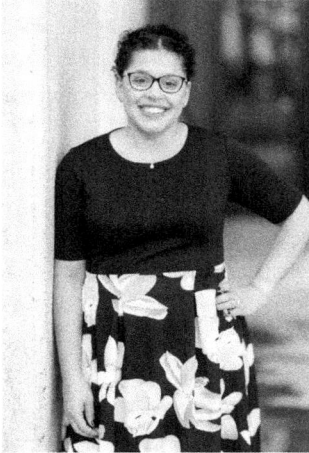

Goal setting has always been a challenging thing for me; perhaps it's an attention deficit or perhaps it's imposter syndrome. One day I read that quote above and it resonated with me deeply, as I hope it does for you. Whether you apply this mindset personally or professionally, I think we are all so much greater than we give ourselves credit for and capable of so much more than we believe.

In 2018 I met a gentleman on a plane and told him about my crazy idea to get more education out into the healthcare industry. Here we are, five years later, with two books, a certificate program, and countless hours of education provided across the country. Many thanks to MGMA for allowing Kem and me to do our part in ushering forward new generations of revenue cycle and finance leaders. Craig, Jeff, Rob, Christy – I could go on because the list is long, as have been our conversations. The leaders at this association are only paralleled in excellence by the conversations we have and the goals we share for this industry.

Thank you to my CEO and friend, Chris Henkenius for believing in me and supporting my crazy ideas for revenue cycle changes during a pandemic while giving me the grace and space to write yet another book. To my co-author and business partner in success, Kem Tolliver, we have worked together longer than either of us would like to mention and we've had so much fun every single day. Thank you to my mentors Nizar Webhi, Laurie Baedke, Nicole Bianchi, Denise Branson, Christine Moheiser, Barbara Miller, and Lavinia Wallace. Past, present, and future, these individuals have had lasting impact on my character, my ethics, and my beliefs. I am only the sum total of my experiences and my experiences with each of you have changed me for the better.

To my children, all of you, whether through birth, marriage, or the fact that you showed up for dinner one night and stayed, thank you for every second of joy you've brought into my life.

Finally, to Travis, it's a strange gift to have someone in your corner who so completely supports you and entertains your silly whims. You laugh at my terrible jokes, keep me stuffed full of the most delicious meals, and genuinely listen to any anecdote I want to tell you (even when it's 3 a.m. and you've heard that pun a hundred times before). Thank you for being my rock, my best friend, my gaming partner, movie watcher, and support system.

My hope is that this book serves as inspiration. That it drives collaborative conversations and, inevitably, that it transforms financial outlooks in a positive way.

—Taya

Kem Tolliver

"In learning you will teach, and in teaching you will learn."

—*Phil Collins*

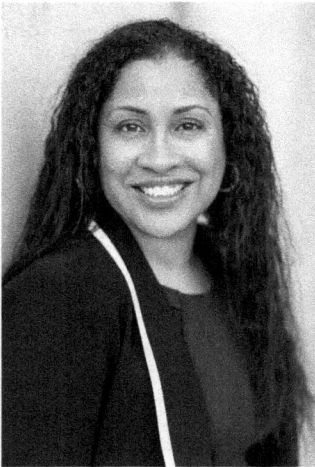

As a child, I loved playing school – cutting puzzles and comics from the Sunday newspaper and making copies of lessons I'd been taught throughout the week. I so looked forward to teaching my class (who were no more than my unwilling siblings, cousins and friends) how to add, read and write in cursive. It's an enormous gift to teach, but there's a greater reward in learning during the experience.

My co-author, my dear friend Taya, and I truly enjoy paying it forward by sharing our knowledge and experiences with you: our healthcare tribe. Our loyalty to the healthcare profession has taken us on a marvelous journey filled with many memories and exciting adventures.

Thank you to the team at Medical Revenue Cycle Specialists: Steve, Tiera, Denise, Monica, Vijay, Jacob, and Nick, for holding down the fort and inspiring me with your commitment to excellence in everything you do, which allows me to pursue authorship and creativity.

To my Ali and Tolliver family, service is ingrained in our DNA. It is an honor to be born an Ali and a blessing to be married into the Tollivers. There's no "award" for planting, feeding, watering, and caring for a wife – but if there was, then Tyrone would have it pinned. To my two-legged children, Tye and Sasha, as well as my four-legged fur babies, Meaty and Luna – you are the center of all good things in my world.

Special appreciation to MGMA for consistently setting the bar high for professional development and certification of healthcare leaders. Thank you for keeping Taya and me on speed dial. We'll keep answering the Bat-Signal.

From those on the front lines to those in cubicles and those working from home – your efforts create the momentum which drives this industry forward. Thank you for your service.

—Kem

Chapter 1

Cost Containment

When we say cost containment, what do we mean? Chances are you're envisioning finding cheaper vendors, trimming staff benefits, and other corporate culture faux pas. What we want you to envision isn't cutting back, trimming the fat, or sacrificing quality for the almighty dollar. We're talking about understanding your costs to the degree that you can confidently say what is necessary, that you are paying what is appropriate for what is necessary, and that you are monitoring for things that will exacerbate cost without benefit to the patient, the practice, or the general population in which you work.

The general public would likely be concerned to know that healthcare leaders intentionally work to contain healthcare costs. This doesn't mean that we are decreasing the value or safety within the care we provide; it means we are ensuring that we have the resources to sustain the services we are providing. We are in the unique position to have portions of our revenue dictated by federal and state regulatory entities. Other portions of our revenue are determined by insurance company formulas – oftentimes with little to no room for negotiation. Our other revenue source is from our customer: the patient. Other industries have a different battle with cost containment. In comparison to the amounts paid (fee schedules) by either our patients or a third party, our costs vary substantially and are often higher than our revenue per encounter. In a healthcare setting, the function of containing cost must be done in

1

a manner that does not jeopardize, but allows for care to continue. In order to fund healthcare innovations, technology, and general overhead costs, we must identify waste in spending by maximizing our containment strategies.

Let's go back to the original question "What is cost containment?" Let's break it down into portions that describe the issue more comprehensively.

Cost containment addresses:

1. How to safely reduce operational cost
2. How to define the total cost of care
3. Optimizing your payvider systems
4. Managing margins realistically
5. Making budgeting processes dynamic
6. Evaluating the variations of costing by site and service

If you're reading this book, the assumption has been made that you've been in this field for a while. You've earned your stripes, so to speak, in the field of revenue cycle. If some terms and phrases seem familiar whereas others seem foreign, use the glossary to help, and dig into other research on these topic areas. That's what we did while putting this book together, and it's amazing what you'll find. With that said, let's unpack the six items above.

1.1 Reducing Operational Cost

This item is first for a reason: any expense reduction equates to a direct revenue boost. Unless, of course, you've reduced expense without intentionality. The word strategy will be used in this book frequently because it's essential that we drive home the importance of intentional thought for each of these sections.

When evaluating potential reductions for operational costs, always consider:

1. The total savings this change will create

2. The impact on operations

3. The implications to patient safety, wellness or access

4. Potential impacts to provider satisfaction or productivity

The first areas to look at are always going to be the biggest areas of spend, because impacts here equate to the biggest return on investment. We recommend starting with five high-cost areas we like to call the "high five":

1. Staffing

2. Salaries & benefits

3. Facility costs

4. Medical supplies

5. Third-party services

Staffing

Before evaluating whether to cut staff, make sure to review the workflows, processes and productivity at your organization. Historically, practices have applied a reactive approach to staff management, but with more data at our disposal, we're able to look at staffing from an evidence-based standpoint.

Evidence shows that having too few employees can result not only in burnout, but also in poor patient satisfaction, reduced levels of care, medical errors, patient attrition, and poorer patient outcomes. Our long-term goal is financial viability of the practice, which cannot be achieved without focusing on the reason we are in business – patient care. Best practice is to evaluate by department with actual data to ascertain needs and risks. Below is an example of what that looks like at a small private practice, Cutten Mend Health, for three departments.

Exhibit 1.1 Cutten Mend Health Department Evaluation

Dept	Financial Impact	Data	Needs	Risk
Front Desk	This department is the first point of interaction with the patient. They are directly responsible for eligibility and benefit verification as well as the accuracy of patient contact information and point-of-care collections for copays, coinsurances, and past-due balances. Current staff = 2	This department takes in 1,500 calls per week System training received once at hire Payer/plan training given once at hire	This department needs the time to enter accurately and effectively Annual system training Quarterly payer/plan updates	Without adequate staffing, this department is at a high risk for inaccurate demographic entry and failure to collect patient responsibilities adequately. Bad data at this position means claim denials, difficulty chasing revenue and lower revenue collected.
Billing Dept	This department manages the claims billing and posting process. Current staff = 1	This biller processes 560 claims per week Only OJT training No interaction with front desk	This department needs more support to work claim denials, appeals, and to properly scrub claims. Employee could benefit from additional training on coding compliance	Without infusing additional training benefits or hiring additional personnel, this department will suffer from burnout, too little time to confirm accurate entry of claims, and poor appeals productivity, leading to revenue decline. Without interaction with the front desk this employee will continue to work through repeated errors of the same type.

Dept	Financial Impact	Data	Needs	Risk
Medical Assistants	This department's responsibility is to take patients back to the exam room, perform and document initial vitals, give shots as ordered, and reset the room for the next patient. Current staff: 7	This department takes back 540 patients per week. Each MA is responsible for approximately 11 patients per day. Processes reviewed indicate significant downtime.	Employees can be cross-trained to help support the calls at the front desk and allow additional time for them to perform improved data entry and patient collections.	There is a great level of animosity between the front desk staff (who have no downtime) and the MAs who have ample downtime. Without cross-training, there is a lack of work balance between departments which creates a cultural challenge.

We aren't going to take you through the whole practice because you get the picture here. The idea is to get a good understanding of what's in place versus what's needed. With further evaluation, it may become clear that the MAs in place are overstaffed, or that there is a need for MAs to adopt additional provider support tasks. The key point is that you should first evaluate the data associated with staffing workflows, productivity and overall impact prior to making cuts in staffing.

To contain costs in this area:

1. Focus on retaining staff by reducing burnout, supporting the needs of staff and ensuring adequate staffing

2. Cross-train employees where applicable, especially between departments that have difficulty working collaboratively

3. Perform training and retraining on critical job functions to ensure peak performance

As you consider strategies for staff cost-reduction, include repeatable and scalable processes that do not negatively impact your operations as your workforce transitions. Importing knowledge from individuals and placing that knowledge into repeatable functions allows for your organization to focus on the process rather than the person. The process can then be customized and tailored to your unique needs and scaled through automation.

Salaries & Benefits

First things first, don't break the law. If you're evaluating cuts to salaries and benefits, it's critical to consult with counsel and human resource experts to make sure you know what you can and can't touch. For example, you can elect to do away with paid time off (PTO), but if you do so, you cannot do away with any time employees have already accrued.

Likewise, you have to retain pay equity without discrimination. You will find that some things are required, like workers' compensation and social security taxes, and that cutting salaried employees' rates below a certain amount may shift them to an hourly classification. Remember, on top of all the above, you must abide by both state and federal laws.

When evaluating staff salaries, look at benchmarks for similar specialties and similarly sized facilities in your geographic area or one that is similar. Just as you did with the staffing assessments, evaluate the potential impacts of reducing salaries. Healthcare salaries and benefits are on the rise, especially post-pandemic. Reducing salaries and benefits could result in staff attrition, high turnover rates and potentially low-quality hires for those turned-over positions. "In its 2016 Human Capital Benchmarking Report, the Society for Human Resource Management estimated that companies spend an average of 42 days to fill a position and $4,129 per hire."[1] In addition, research shows it can take anywhere from six months to two years for a new hire to reach a break-even in terms of productivity and overall performance.

To be clear, you should still review staffing, salaries and benefits. Review multiple vendors for health insurance, employment assistance programs, and the cost of other benefit programs to identify whether there are vendors that are a better fit for your organization. Just keep in mind that these cost reduction methods can end up costing more in the long run if you aren't careful.

To contain costs in this area:

1. Look at benchmarks for salaries and benefits and compare to your own expenses

2. Be mindful of the costs of staff attrition and rehire expenses

3. Look at other vendors and lower-cost benefits for employees

Lower-cost benefits can include[2]:

1. Offering vision and dental with the health plan

2. Offering high-deductible health plans

3. Providing flexible employee schedules or non-standard schedules (four ten-hour days, etc.) where possible

4. Allow administrative staff to work from home – this can result in other savings and higher productivity

5. Quarterly movie tickets – for a staff of 25 this may cost roughly $300 total, depending on your area

6. Monthly lunch – this can be done relatively inexpensively, but the perceived value to employees is high

7. Employee discounts – many companies offer employee discounts for corporations (cable companies, tech companies, etc.) and offering these to employees can sometimes be a no-cost benefit

8. Paid VTO – allows employees to give back to the community in ways that matter to them and also indicates that leadership cares about what is of interest to employees

Facility Expenses

The largest facility expense is typically that of renting space, which brings us back, yet again, to strategy. Leases and building purchases are long-term expenses and should be planned with significant focus and intention. Decreasing facility expenses is challenging to do between renewal years, so it is imperative that you are aware of your lease terms and renewal dates. Review your agreement and identify:

7

1. The lease term (length)

2. The termination options and notification dates for renewal and non-renewal

3. Renewal options (if any exist)

When you have opportunities to discuss rate negotiations, come prepared. Know the going rate for commercial space and don't make threats/ultimatums you aren't willing to back up. Moving a practice is expensive, so ensure that the benefit outweighs the risk before you threaten non-renewal of the lease.

When you own the building, you may have more options to decrease facility expense, for example:

- Regular maintenance – this will help prohibit leaks, higher heating/cooling expenses, and damage from rodents and other environmental hazards.
- High-quality HVAC and filter changes – this will keep your employees healthier and drive increased efficiency of your HVAC.
- Reduce off-hours use – if your facility is only open for a portion of the day or portion of the week, implement smart technology to minimize the utilization of heating/cooling and electricity.

Whether you lease or own, you can also encourage staff to shut down their computers on Friday afternoon, power off printers that aren't needed, and turn off waiting room televisions. These small things add up and can be easily integrated into the closing workflow for staff.

Another area of significant expense is insurance coverage. Clinical space is going to be rated differently than administrative/clerical space. If you have these areas clearly defined, you can reduce expense with your workers' compensation and general liability carriers by rating these areas separately based on their square footage. Keep in mind that if you reorganize the facility, it will be your responsibility to inform the carrier of changes.

Medical Supplies

The best way to reduce the cost of medical supplies is through proper supply chain management (SCM). SCM is a significant undertaking, but makes a huge impact on overall organizational expenses and performance. SCM is the umbrella for several other important components of oversight which are each essential for success:

- Product management
- Utilization oversight
- Vendor/supplier management
- Inventory management

Product Management

Before you can begin managing the supplies you need and how to procure them, you must understand what your facility needs. There are several ways to determine the supplies needed by each facility, but the most common approach is to review supplies by the services provided. To get started:

1. Pull a list of the supplies ordered over the last 12-24 months and sort by unit quantity

2. Categorize supplies into two sections:

   a. Standard expenses – This will include items used for every visit like hand sanitizer, table paper, and gloves

   b. Service or department-related expenses – This will be specific by service or department. For example: hyaluronic acid injectables may be allocated to rheumatology or to specific procedures where that injectable is given

3. Document the quantity still on hand for each supply item by type

4. Pull a list of the procedures/services performed over the same time period by frequency and categorize them by level of use (e.g. high-use, low-use, etc.). The way you label your categories should fit your use of this report.

Once done, your report will look something like this:

Exhibit 1.2 Product Management Example

Product	Use Type	Dept./ Service	Ordered last 12 months	Quantity on Hand (QOH)	Rate of Use
Gloves – M	Standard	All	150 boxes	7 boxes	High
Table Paper	Standard	All	50 rolls	40 rolls	High
Flu Vaccine	Service	Flu Season	550 vials	200 vials	Annual

Reviewing this sheet gives you benchmarks for what the practice orders regularly and what they use regularly. For example, you can see in the table above that in the last 12 months, the practice ordered 150 boxes of size medium gloves. There are only 7 boxes on hand, which indicates an average monthly utilization of approximately 12 boxes. This information will help you set par levels for this standard item.

The report also identifies a significant over-purchase of table paper and flu vaccine. This indicates that though these are being used and should remain on the product list, they should be further evaluated for utilization rate.

While reviewing, you may also find that you have products you are unable to tie back to a service or regular need; in that case you should dig in with your providers and department leads to identify why those products were ordered.

Before you wrap this report, discuss with staff to identify product needs. Are there items that you typically don't have when you need them or items for which providers have been asking? This isn't part of cost containment but can be part of revenue enhancement if the items relate to billable services.

Once the report is completed, look at the items that can be standardized as well to eliminate variation – reduced variation can reduce cost.

Utilization Oversight

Now that you have identified the products being ordered, review products that are:

1. High-cost: Negotiating these items with vendors can help reduce the expense of costly supplies

2. High-use: Negotiating these items with vendors, even for small savings, can quickly add up to large savings overall

3. Outliers: Review areas where the amounts purchased don't align to the services rendered and adjust par levels as needed to contain supply costs

4. Rate of Reimbursement: Because some medical supply costs are billable, pull a report of injectables (for instance) and compare that against the quantities ordered and quantities which remain to identify areas where the cost of the medication may not have been negated by reimbursement

Vendor/Supplier Management

You should now have a good understanding of what products your facility needs, how often, and why. Use this information to inform strategic discussions with vendors/suppliers. Make sure to take advantage of Group Purchasing Organizations (GPOs) or other member savings that exist. For example, several associations including MGMA, have supply savings programs that members can take advantage of. This type of supply savings is offered by organizations with a national presence as a member benefit. Participation in a GPO is a strategy used to leverage volume-based discounts for supplies and approved services. The discounts are shared amongst GPO members by leveraging economies of scale. Types of supplies and services that may be purchased via a GPO include insurance, medical supplies, clerical supplies, and document-management supplies.

Evaluate multiple vendors whenever you review supply prices, but remember that the biggest savings present when long-term vendor relationships have been established. Establish your product supply list as your core supply list and negotiate prices for all of them. Be careful that reductions made to certain supplies aren't offset by the vendor by increasing the cost of other high-use supplies.

Inventory Management

Knowing what you have, what's getting low and what's needed is the genesis of inventory management. For example, you may know that you have 10 boxes of large gloves, but you may not know whether that quantity is sufficient. That comes down to understanding frequency of use. For every item you purchase you should have par levels set.

Exhibit 1.3 Par Level

Item	Quantity on Hand	Par Level	Quantity Needed
Gloves – Large, Latex Free	10 boxes	9 boxes	0
Gloves – Medium, Latex Free	7 boxes	15 boxes	8 boxes
Gloves – Small, Latex Free	3 boxes	3 boxes	0

In the above table, the clinic has created a spreadsheet with the par levels set for each item. The clinical manager reviews biweekly and places orders based on what is needed to bring the organization to par level inventory. This example is very basic; it is likely you will want to include other fields such as supplier, item number, alternate suppliers/item numbers, time to delivery, etc. Time to delivery can be essential for items that are regularly backordered or challenging to obtain. In some cases, you may want to increase your par level to accommodate for that challenge in the supply chain.

Once you have combined product management, utilization oversight, vendor/supplier management, and inventory management, you should be able to create a regular routine of review and evaluation to help contain medical supply costs.

Third-Party Services

More often than ever before, third-party vendors are establishing fees as a percentage of revenue as opposed to a flat fee. To contain costs of third-party service suppliers, closely review your agreements. When you navigate into percentage-based agreements, your goal may be a zero-risk arrangement, where the supplier does not get paid if you don't. This is a thorny road, however, as it increases the incentive for the supplier to get paid. In zero-risk agreements you will want to maintain a significant amount of oversight to verify that there are no instances of improper behavior.

When it comes to using third-party services, it is critically important to remember that, regardless of any contract terms, you will most likely be responsible for things like:

- Delivering patient records in a timely manner upon request
- Protecting and maintaining patient records within regulatory guidelines

Keep in mind that having a third-party agreement does not automatically mean that all the components in that agreement will be enforceable. For example, the Office of Civil Rights (OCR) began their Right of Access Initiative in 2019, mandating patient access to records within specific timelines. Many third-party records companies work to provide this service for practices and facilities, and most contracts state that they will be responsible to provide that information in a timely fashion. However, ultimately the provider practice/facility is responsible for fulfilling the patient's records request in a timely fashion. Likewise, many states have laws that allow providers to bill patients for requested records. The Right of Access Initiative states that facilities may charge a small, reasonable fee for providing a copy of PHI and that the fee billed may only cover the cost of creating the copied record. They go on to note, "this fee is not allowed to include any other associated costs, even if other costs appear to be authorized by state law."[3]

Whenever you consider implementing the services of a third party, make sure you fully understand the implications at the federal and state level should the third party fail to meet regulations or requirements. In addition, remember that the burden of oversight falls to the practice, and take that responsibility seriously to avoid potentially challenging and costly situations.

Achieving Success

Success in reducing operational expenses comes down to planning, execution, and ongoing evaluation. Reviewing ways to optimize staffing, salaries/benefits, facility expenses, medical supplies and third-party services creates the foundation of cost-containment activities.

To succeed with cost containment, you will need to:

1. Annually, review expenses with evaluation of expenses for improvement opportunities
2. Monthly (or more frequently), assess inventory and ordering
3. Quarterly, use cost to contract evaluations to confirm you aren't being billed more than you've negotiated
4. Evaluate processes and workflows for opportunities to minimize expenses where possible (minimization of effort or reduction of resource use)
5. Include cost initiatives in staff success conversations – how your team can help to keep costs low
6. Develop internal controls to mitigate supply theft, over-time, etc.
7. Utilize technology to track, monitor and report

There are many people involved in cost-containment success:

1. Leadership team
   a. Individuals authorized to negotiate and/or sign agreements
   b. Department leaders with significant understanding of team workflows and resource utilization

   c. Managers responsible for inventory, ordering, time keeping, paycheck approvals, etc.

   d. General staff who work in each position have the best insight into workflows and methods that exist today and how they may differ from documented or perceived workflows and protocols:

      i. Direct and indirect departments staff – if you are reviewing, for example, a workflow variation for intake staff that has resulted in significant overtime, also obtain workflow information from other departments who interact with the intake staff. This will help to identify if responsibilities are being shifted to the wrong department, if the root cause of the work overflow is initiating from a different department, etc.

Focus on Communication

Staff should be aware that there are new ongoing strategies for the long-term viability of the organization. Without clear communication, expense reduction efforts may create confusion for staff. For example, if you are switching medical supply vendors, explain this to staff who are used to interacting closely with their former vendor representative.

Though this is business, it's likely they've formed a kinship with those individuals and will not otherwise understand why the decision has been made. As usually occurs, the imagination is often worse than reality. So, a lack of transparency may indicate to staff that the organization is not on solid footing. Keep staff informed at an appropriate level, to keep them engaged in the cost-containment process and focused on their job instead of speculation.

Technology and Operational Expense

Optimal use of technology can be one of the greatest ways to optimize cost. You can use automated processes to speed up workflows and, in turn, reduce staff hours. Convert patients to electronic billing where possible to reduce the expense of paper billing. Increase utilization of the patient portal to obtain patient forms and documents before visits to reduce the work required by intake staff, the postage of mailing forms, or the cost of providers getting behind due to late intake.

Some frequently overlooked areas to optimize include:

- Supply chain management
- Optimization of collections processes before outsourcing
- Use of electronic scheduling and confirmation services
- Templates that vary by service/department
- Use of a practice management system for resource management
- Analytics tools that indicate revenue leaks

1.2 Total Cost of Care

Defining Total Cost of Care

The CMS Office of the Actuary publishes the National Health Expenditure (NHE) report containing data that healthcare financial leaders should track to understand the current and projected state of healthcare spending. The data shown within this report sets the tone for the manner in which CMS and other healthcare payers will address their spending. The NHE showed that in 2020, healthcare expenses represented 19.7% of total Gross Domestic Product (GDP). As expected, due to the decrease in healthcare services output during the COVID-19 Public Health Emergency, spending declined from $417.6 billion in 2020 to $286.8 billion. The NHE projects a 5.1% growth in the health share of GDP between 2021 and 2030. During 2020, the United Kingdom's health share of GDP was 12.8%. The comparison of the US and the UK shows the US with a 6.9% elevated health share of GDP.[4]

The current rate of healthcare spending has been a significant driver of total cost of care reduction methodologies. There must be an evolution in the manner in which healthcare spending is managed for long-term sustainability. The total cost of care model prioritizes the analysis of healthcare spending in episodes of care over certain periods of time in a variety of settings. It also takes into account direct and indirect costs of care, which are necessary as they serve as key factors in the total cost of care. Oversight of direct and indirect healthcare costs helps to manage overall healthcare spending costs. Understanding these costs and each point of elevation promotes the ability to manage and reduce these costs through efficiencies and supportive services.

Exhibit 1.4 Direct and Indirect Household Health Costs[5]

Direct Healthcare Costs	Indirect Healthcare Costs
Primary care and specialist services	Food expenses that are above and beyond typical food
Health and supplemental insurance premiums	Housing and shelter
Prescription and non-prescription drugs	Transportation
Rehabilitation services (occupational, speech, physical)	Technology, internet and other communications
Hospitalization	Permanent or temporary disability due to illness of patient or family member
Surgical services	Patient or family employment changes
Durable medical equipment	Location changes due to illness of patient or family member

The total cost of care ties together our need to manage costs with our funding sources' need to do the same. Payers have officially moved away from utilizing fee-for-service as the only payment methodology so they can contain their costs. The traditional fee-for-service model now incorporates elements of value-based programs, pay for performance, and risk-based payments, which all align with the state and federal objective of healthcare cost-containment. In addition to healthcare spending reduction, total cost of care initiatives seek to create a healthier population by increasing the quality of care in order to improve patient outcomes. These initiatives are being achieved when CMS partners with stakeholders such as states, who then partner with community providers. Community providers are key to making this payment model work, as they have direct access to patients and are usually the gatekeepers to keeping patients in care. Total Cost of Care models eliminate working in silos and instead offer financial incentives to collaborate in efforts to track quality and illness burdens as well as to reduce costs, inefficiencies and overuse.

The Total Cost of Care model originated from the "Maryland All-Payer Model," which expired on December 31, 2018. The All-Payer model allowed the state to create quality and outcomes that improved population health while limiting outpatient and hospital costs for Medicare beneficiaries. This model worked relatively well for hospitals as they worked around the clock to reduce hospital-acquired conditions and preventable hospital readmissions. The latter objective was a challenge, because while hospitals had the internal infrastructure to coordinate their efforts to achieve the outlined Medicare metrics for the program, they lacked the necessary coordination with community physicians to meet the unnecessary readmissions metrics.

The Total Cost of Care model was built to incorporate assistance and financial resources for hospital systems to coordinate with community physicians to meet shared goals. One key metric for success with the Total Cost of Care model is to limit hospital cost growth to 3.58% per capita. The other important metric is for Maryland hospitals to save the Medicare program $300 million annually by the conclusion of 2023. Other metrics include[6]:

- Care will be coordinated across both hospital and non-hospital settings, including mental health and long-term care.
- The model will invest resources in patient-centered care teams and primary care enhancements.
- Maryland will set a range of quality and care improvement goals. Providers will be paid more when patient outcomes are better.
- Maryland will set a range of hospital quality, care transformation, and population health goals as part of the Statewide Integrated Health Improvement Strategy.[7]
- State flexibility will facilitate programs centered on the unique needs of Marylanders, the provider community, geographic settings, and other key demographics.

Measuring and calculating the total cost of care can be improved by using metrics that impact healthcare costs. Use the table below to internally assess the ways that certain factors will impact operational and healthcare expenses.

Exhibit 1.5 Healthcare Metrics

Metric	Description	Use Case
Patient Demographics	Age, gender, home address, employment status	Unique identifiers and status of beneficiary receiving care
Type of Service	Inpatient, outpatient, emergency room, E/M, procedures	Allows for further description of required claim usage (UB -04 or 837) and payment rules
Diagnosis Related Group (DRG)	Inpatient diagnosis group	Tracks and reports payments for related diagnoses and services
Diagnosis Codes	Description of medical illness being treated	Describes acute and chronic illnesses. Demonstrates risk of morbidity.
Date of Service / Begin and End Date	Date that healthcare services were rendered. Date of onset.	Used to capture and track average length of stay
Place of Service	Location that services were rendered	Validates where services were provided to allow for accurate selection of place of service code and use of appropriate billing rules
HCPCS / CPT	Service or procedure code that describes the type of service rendered to beneficiary	Notification of services performed by a provider and facility
Modifier	Code added to CPT/ HCPCS	Alters original service type and provides additional description
Length of Stay	First, subsequent and discharge of beneficiary's hospital stay for related condition	Measures length of hospitalization with benchmarks for similar hospitalizations
Provider	Clinician who rendered services for patient attributed to them by CMS; using their NPI #	Uses taxonomy code to indicate specialty for correct claims processing
Allowed Amount	Contracted amount paid by insurance for services rendered	Tracks reimbursement in comparison to billed amount and contractual adjustments

As mentioned previously, collaboration is a critical component to the success of a Total Cost of Care model. CMS created the Centers for Medicare and Medicaid Innovation (CMMI) to support "the development and testing of innovative health care payment and service delivery models."[8] Within the umbrella of CMMI, Care Transformation Organizations (CTOs) were funded to offer no-cost transformation, interoperability and care collaboration between community physicians and hospitals. Under the Maryland Total Cost of Care (MD TCOC) model, physician practices have access to CTOs who have the knowledge and funding to assist them in achieving necessary program measures. The 2021 modified Stark Law and Anti-Kickback statutes also assist with allowing hospital systems to financially support community physicians when they are jointly working toward shared savings through collaborative participation in value-based or risk-based programs. These CTOs range from medical societies, Managed Services Organizations (MSOs), hospitals and other approved health systems.

Maryland CTOs are paid to provide care coordination and practice transformation support to primary care physicians; again – at no cost to the practice. Why primary care physicians, you ask? Let's consider what we've discussed so far with TCOC. The metric within TCOC that could be directly managed outside of the hospital is reduction of preventable hospital readmissions. This metric is square on the backs of primary care physicians (PCPs). They are the true gatekeepers and patient engagement specialists in the care continuum. It's no surprise that CMMI is charging PCPs with this responsibility. In a step forward from the original "All Payer Model" that only financially incentivized hospitals, the MD TCOC model now includes the Maryland Primary Care Program (MD PCP) which provides performance-based payments to PCPs. The CTOs receive a percentage of the care management fee for each PCP practice it assists with transformation under the MD PCP program.

Other key stakeholders within the MD TCOC model are state-based agencies whose goals are to improve population health outcomes and manage healthcare costs. As Maryland continues to participate in innovative CMS payment models, the necessity for state-based organizations to manage, guide, collaborate and track progress with these initiatives is essential.

1.3 Payvider Systems

Acronyms have become customary in healthcare, and as that continues, we welcome the use of a relatively new term, "payvider." Contrary to most other terms in our industry, this word explains itself right in its name: payer + provider = payvider.

According to RevCycle Intelligence,

"A payvider is a provider organization that operates its own health plans. But the payvider model also includes other risk-based collaborations between payers and providers, such as direct employment of physicians by large payers, joint ventures or long-term risk-based contracts, and payers partnering with entrants."[9]

If that doesn't break it down enough, take, for example, risk-based Medicare Advantage payment models. The collaboration of payer and provider in these models is defined as a payvider system and they are increasingly popular. The popularity of the payvider system continues to rise as the need to integrate quality care with financial risk becomes more prevalent. According to Becker's Healthcare, "The ability to control providers' delivery and payment of care has many competitive advantages. However, by no means is success guaranteed."[10]

In this section we are going to review:

1. The role that payvider systems play in cost reduction
2. Examples of current payvider systems
3. Risk vs. reward – finding the balance
4. The role and impact of coders on payvider systems

Payvider systems can be very complex and require significant oversight to be successful. If structured properly, though, they can be more than worth the effort.

The Role Payvider Systems Play in Cost Reduction

The structure of payvider systems is varied, as is the proportion of risk between payer and provider. The goals of a payvider system will include high-touch, member-centered care for a more appropriate system and benefit utilization, thereby reducing the cost to the industry. As such, they require a significant amount of dedication to collaboration, with both sides playing an essential role in the likelihood for success. According to Becker's Hospital Review, "In February 2021, the Banner|Aetna plan announced a long-term agreement to extend its joint venture relationship, citing an average cost savings of 8%-14%, improved member experiences, and growth to approximately 350,000 members."[11]

Average savings in the double-digits along with significant growth in membership is a huge win for Aetna, and these successes result in notable rewards for Banner as well. Deep-diving into the reports, you will find that the savings seen by Banner|Aetna were due mostly to pharmacy-related savings through medication-management programs and waste-reduction programs. It's clear why these are areas of success that Aetna would not have been able to achieve without Banner Health.

The provider's role in guiding patients' medication plans, encouraging compliance, and adhering to the insurer's formularies are pivotal steps that must be taken at the provider level. The creation/negotiation of prescription formularies and streamlining the prescriptive authorization process are critical steps that must be done at the payer level. So, both parties are essential to success with this program.

The Payvider Approach

1. Payers
    a. Use data they have access to in order to identify areas of potential cost savings, for example: high use of costly procedures, services, or medications

    b. Define the opportunity of cost savings and what "success" means from a dedicated improvement program

    c. Offer a portion of cost savings to providers who are willing to try to achieve them in the form of a risk-based agreement

2. Providers

    a. Take a clinical approach to reviewing the areas of potential cost savings

    b. Work alongside payers to identify strategies which can achieve cost savings

    c. Agree to accept a portion of risk in exchange for the possibility of receiving a portion of the cost saved by the payer in the form of a bonus

Types of Payvider Systems

There are three types of payvider systems:

1. Payers who branch into the provider space
2. Providers who branch into the payer space
3. Joint ventures between payers and providers who don't want to branch into other areas of expertise

Joint ventures are becoming more prevalent, including the example of Banner|Aetna which brought together an enormous network of providers with a vast network of coverage, providing more choices, resources, and benefits for over 250,000 patients.[12]

Risk vs. Reward – Finding the Balance

Any collaborative agreement comes with elements of risk, and the same holds true for payvider systems. In order to reduce cost, it's critical that providers are selective about risk-based agreements. The opportunity for great bonuses is wonderful, but to reach them the goals must be achievable and cannot cost more to implement than could potentially be realized by the reward structure. Review three areas to determine your readiness to accept risk:

1. **Know Your Community**. You will need to forecast the likelihood of success to determine if you have a risk worth taking. For this reason, forecasts are essential, but they require an accurate picture of the community you serve – demographics, social determinant of health (SDoH) barriers, disease trends and prevalence, etc.

2. **Define What You Are Responsible For.** If you were in a class, you'd refer to the rubric. Payvider systems work the same way: you need to know what you're being graded on. You don't want to spend all your efforts reducing hospital readmissions only to find out you're being graded on reduced medication abandonment. You have to know what you will be responsible for to make sure that those goals are realistic and appropriate.

3. **Utilization and Care Management** – Most payvider systems will require an element of utilization review and care management at some level because they have both been proven as effective cost reduction methods when implemented properly. If your practice/facility doesn't have strong success in these areas, you will want to review how they impact your ability to succeed in a risk-based payment model.

According to Guidehouse Insights in 2021, the most successful payvider systems are those that start with integrated scorecards so that payers and providers succeed or fail together. For example:

Exhibit 1.6 Playbook for Payvider Collaboration[13]

	From Traditional, Brinksmanship, Zero-Sum Negotiations with Opposed Goals (Traditional Managed Care Playbook)	To Strategically, Financially, and Operationally Aligned Scorecards that Put Members First
Payer Metrics	• Membership • MLR • ALR	• No. 1 or No. 2 market share in terms of both members and share of wallet • Stable 3%-5% operating margin

From Traditional, Brinksmanship, Zero-Sum Negotiations with Opposed Goals (Traditional Managed Care Playbook)		To Strategically, Financially, and Operationally Aligned Scorecards that Put Members First
	• Provider Discount of Charges • STARS Score • Risk Score	• Lower medical cost trend per beneficiary vs. market • 6%-8% ALR "best practice" (all in) • 80%-85% MLR "best practice"
Provider Metrics	• IP Market Share • Volumes • Cost/Case • Managed Care Contract Yield (1-Discount)	• Commercial Reimbursement Rates: Up to 150% of MCR; MA and MCD, 100% MCR • 20% of fees at risk, with 10% bonus upside • Purchaser, patient, member, physician net promoter score > 30 (scale of -100 to +100) • Mutual penalities/rebates for underperformance

Notably, payvider systems are not a one-size-fits-all model. Of the top five areas projected to have the greatest growth potential, three are on the East Coast. Meanwhile, of the top five highest performing areas, eighty percent are in California. Other community factors matter, like access to care, cost, utilization, and quality.[14]

The Role and Impact of Coders on Payvider Systems

Demonstrating illness complexity within a population is a key component to making risk and reimbursement determinations within the payvider model. Patients with complex conditions can be challenging outliers when evaluating the rest of the community demographics you serve. Identifying complex cases can help:

(1) explain certain unavoidable high costs

(2) help define patients who should be assigned to care management programs

(3) justify larger payments for certain patients

Coders play a very important role in the identification of complex cases because they are the ones evaluating the diagnosis and hierarchical condition categories (HCCs) of the patients seen at your facility.

Each individual beneficiary has a unique condition, co-morbidities and SDOH. Utilizing certified coders to extract proper specificity of coding based on provider documentation is a critical component in ensuring success of a payvider model. In many programs, reimbursements are increased/decreased based on the HCCs; for this reason, it is essential that coders and managers have accurate HCC data to review.

An example of increased/decreased reimbursement would be based on the ICD-10-CM or diagnosis code selection for a patient population. The diagnosis appended to each encounter will create a risk group that will be incorporated into a Risk Adjustment Factor (RAF). This RAF is used to forecast and project payments for a patient population under each provider's care. Encounter documentation that lacks "meat" will not support higher projected payments for a highly complex patient population. Certified coders have a keen eye for detail, and when a proper HCC program is put in place, coders are essential in applying the correct diagnosis code that fully explains the complexity and medical decision making required to manage chronic illnesses.

The level of detail offered by coders will allow for the justification of a higher RAF, thereby allowing a payvider to accurately project future spending. This accuracy will in turn justify a higher rate of reimbursement if warranted. Coders are also responsible for ensuring clinical documentation integrity by educating healthcare providers on clinical documentation improvement (CDI) rules to ensure compliance. Having a certified coder as part of your team will give your organization the advantage of having professionals who are adept at communicating billing improvement opportunities with physicians and capturing appropriate receivable amounts. The communications between coders and physicians are more collegial than that of routine support staff, as coders must maintain CEUs to keep their certifications. This requires them to engage in routine professional development in their areas of expertise.

Integrating certified coders if you don't already have them on staff can appear to be purely a cost increase; however, there is significant opportunity cost without coders. Carefully evaluate the benefits of a payvider model and the contributions of certified coders to your organization's performance to payvider system goals.

1.4 Margin Management

When describing the margins for a business, think of the concept as profits after expenses have been deducted from revenues. Margins can be calculated by subtracting total cost from net revenue. Margins may be expressed in dollar amounts (e.g., $10,000 margin), by percentage (e.g., 25% margin), or by return on investment (e.g., ROI = Net Income/ Investment Cost). The higher the margins, the better an organization is performing financially.

The healthcare industry has unique margin management challenges. In other industries, there is a level of control over revenues by setting rates and collecting upon those exact rates. In this model, the process of margin management is somewhat straightforward. In healthcare, providers of care do not control rate-setting. We establish charge amounts, but our funding sources (insurance companies) set our payment rates (allowable amounts) as well as the payment rules – which are complex and ever changing.

Prioritizing margin management is an essential component of financial management to measure how successful we are in our financial efforts. As such, financial leaders are on the hunt for strategies to improve margins. Oftentimes, the low-hanging fruit in margin management is workforce reduction. Don't get me wrong; workforce oversight is a great way to identify margin barriers, but we may shoot ourselves in the foot if we attempt to decrease staffing without research as a form of margin management. When it comes to modeling staffing, we want to be sure that resources are allocated appropriately, all staff are working to their top-performing skill level, no individual has a higher workload than another, and there is an even mix of automation and manual processes. Prior to adding staff to the chopping block, we can right-size our staffing by performing staff allocation reviews.

During the process of conducting a staff allocation analysis, one will want to determine appropriate staffing ratios to work functions, volumes and responsibilities. Determine cost per position and whether certain providers or duties require more resources than others – if so, ensure current staffing levels are right-sized, meaning not under- or overstaffed. Some physicians require more hand-holding and support than others – in these instances, we should readjust staff output expectations to take into consideration unanticipated performance variances. There are also outliers with insurance complexity. Billers assigned to Medicare may require more time interpreting payment rules, filing appeals and checking claim status than those staffers who are assigned to less complicated or lower-volume funding sources.

Cross-training staff to perform the responsibilities of others who might be temporarily pulled in another direction (which happens quite regularly in healthcare facilities) is a great resource for margin management. Determining appropriate pay scales based on performance, tenure, and market trends will provide an equitable compensation structure that takes into consideration key factors of margin management.

Exhibit 1.7 Staff Allocation Matrix

Employee	Status	Hourly Rate	Position	Cross Trained & Cert for Admin & Clinical	Assignment
Ava Avery	FTE	$20.00	Front Desk	Y	Dr. Walls
Sidney Cole	FTE	$23.00	Med Assistant	N	Dr. Jones
Luke Jones	PT	$24.00	Med Assistant	Y	Dr. Walls
Sam Klump	1099	$25.00	Biller	N	Medicare
Tasha Moore	1099	$25.00	Biller	N	BCBS
Zoe Smith	FTE	$18.00	Front Desk	Y	Dr. Jones

Healthcare is a business and our patients are consumers. Whether they pay for their own services out-of-pocket, use employer-paid insurance, or have another funding source, they are revenue-generating for our organizations. Although healthcare is a service industry, we may track and manage our margins by leveraging formulas based on patient care services. Ultimately, the techniques used to deliver care must be taken into consideration for financial modeling.

Since there is an expense to providing care to each patient, we have the ability to analyze these costs using formulas that provide calculations for positive or negative margins. The below margin formulas may be used to track, trend, set and manage organizational margins for pre-determined timeframes. Monthly and annual tracking is common; however, alternative timeframes should be taken into consideration based on your organization's needs.

Exhibit 1.8 Margin Formulas

Margin	Formula (Month or Annual)
Net Profit Margin	Revenue − Expenses ÷ Revenue
Staff Salary Rate by Patient	Total Salary (with or without benefits) ÷ Total # of patients
Gross fee-for-service Revenue	Gross Revenue ÷ Total # of patients
Total Expense	Total Expenses ÷ Total # of patients
Total Medicare Shared Savings Payment (MSSP)	$50 x Total # of patients

Margin Management Framework

Forecasting the fluctuation of profit margins assists with preparing for times that revenues might take a hit – this could occur during the summer months when vacations are taking place or when spikes in communicable diseases such as COVID-19 occur; both may decrease patient and elective service volumes. Maintaining stability with recurring expenses provides a buffer during profit shortfalls.

The information, data, risk and equation for profit margins will differ based on the operation, cost center or area of impact – all will share certain elements and portions of formula development. Goals, outcomes and risks will vary based on the profit margin area. For example, fee-for-service payer reimbursement margins will be based on factors such as contracted rates, staff's ability to collect on accounts, payment posting and other revenue velocity factors. Value-based program participation profit margins will be determined by quality measure and related scoring abilities.

There will be risks to margin goals that will need to be considered and interrupted. Several risks include:

- Injectable/drug cost equal to or greater than service delivery margin
- Technician salary equal to or greater than procedure volume
- Equipment cost compared to testing reimbursement

Organizations' margin goals or profitability goals will be expressed through a margin management framework. Within your margin management framework, you'll want to forecast your profitability goals. These goals will vary based on the area being observed or managed. Utilize a margin management framework to identify margins, current standards, future goals, risks and control strategies.

Exhibit 1.9 Margin Management Framework

Area of Impact	Current Output	Goal	Control Strategy
Staffing	$50,000 per month	Decrease overtime by 25%	Staff allocation analysis
Disparate Software Platforms	$3,750 per month	$2,000 per month	Technology stack audit and integration
Supplies	$6,500 per month	$4,000 per month	Automated inventory control, group purchasing agreement
Commercial Payer Reimbursement	80% of Medicare Allowable	150% of Medicare	Fee schedule analysis and rate negotiations
Benefits & Insurance	10% of Annual Salaries	25% Reduction	Audit current coverage, usage and ROI

In our industry, higher service prices do not always translate to higher profit margins, especially using a fee-for-service reimbursement model. We can manage profits through cost control, data visibility, effective resource allocation, technology optimization, fixing broken processes, and creating a culture of profit prioritization at all levels. Rather than mailing a patient statement, which drops the profit margin, educate staff and collect at the time of service or offer electronic payment options. Many times, we have assumptions about profits without the data to back these assumptions up. Extract data to analyze profit margins and determine margin growth opportunities. Weed out margin risks and address them head on. Prepare for and manage margin reduction by tracking margins in a "cost-center" model. Larger organizations utilize cost-centers for cost and budgeting purposes. Utilize this same approach for margin management.

1.5 Budget Savings

There are many factors that go into how we structure our budgeting process, and that in itself can create savings. In this section we are going to dive into dynamic budgeting, rolling forecasts, saving malpractice expenses and public contributions to organizational expense.

Dynamic Budgeting

Most of us think of the budgeting process as something static. Once the budget is done for the year, it's laminated, placed behind glass and hung next to the Mona Lisa. Thank goodness it's done and now we can avoid doing another of those horribly annoying budgets until next year, right? The challenge with a static budget is that our practices are not static. They evolve, things change, and our budget has to reflect that. In 2020 none of us were prepared for the budget we'd need to have, because none of us were prepared for a global-scale pandemic.

A dynamic budget allows for agility throughout the year. Sadly, a dynamic budget cannot predict a pandemic, but it can provide you with the flexibility needed to make decisions quickly and effectively.

Exhibit 1.10 Static vs. Dynamic Budget Types

Budget Type	Definition	Fit	Effort
Static	This type of budget is finalized once prepared and does not change throughout the year. Think of this like your crockpot meal prepared first thing in the morning for later that evening. Just set it and leave it be.	If your practice is operating with a highly predictable set of circumstances that rarely sees any change throughout the years, this method likely works for you just fine.	Moderate – static budgets are much simpler to complete because they account for one set of circumstances at a minute level.
Dynamic	This type of budget is more fluid; it can adapt to changes in your practice. Think of this type of budget like a dinner party without a fluid guest list. You may need to prepare in advance to know how to shake up the menu a few times as the RSVPs and dietary restrictions flow in.	If your practice sees variations in quantities of visits, changes in services offered, rapid growth, expansion, ancillary service offerings, etc., then you probably want to work with a budget that can grow with you like this one.	High – dynamic budgets are complex and require the evaluation of multiple potentialities at a high level.

To be clear here, a dynamic budget doesn't mean a daily project. A dynamic budget means that you prepare, in advance, for all potential situations. This makes dynamic budgeting extremely complex and time-consuming, but more efficient. The benefit of using a dynamic budget is three-fold:

1. Updated forecasts throughout the year negate the tedious months-long process of static budget creation

2. The updates keep you directionally correct with your long-term strategic plans

3. They retain usefulness and appropriateness much longer than static budgets during the year

Real Impact: The Cost-Savings of Dynamic Budgeting

OSF Healthcare transitioned to dynamic budgeting across all of their hospital locations after a successful two-site pilot program. The results of their full-scale rollout were impressive. According to Healthcare Finance News, "The system has saved $1 million on overall budgeting efforts, with those resources redeployed to higher-value financial planning. There has also been a 75% reduction in the time that's spent on the budget, freeing up about 20,000 hours of leadership time." According to OSF, the shift not only provided cost savings in budgeting efforts and leadership time, but it also allowed for more frequent accountability reviews, progress checks, and earlier intervention to financial challenges.[15]

Rolling Forecasts

A rolling forecast can help you to anticipate costs on an ongoing basis by using historical data to predict upcoming expenses. Whether you are using your accounting management system, a third-party software or Excel, a rolling expense forecast should be in your toolbox for optimal financial management.

Steps to successful rolling forecasts:

1. Identify what you want to review: in this case we will assume we are looking at expenses
2. Determine the timeframe and increments:
   a. Timeframe: Often a 13-month or 25-month lookback is used and can be very helpful for forecasting seasonal variance
   b. Increments: Given the above we'd want to look at the data by month or by quarter; however, if we wanted 60 months of historical data in our rolling forecast, perhaps we'd want to view this by year
3. Key participants: As with all projects, the individuals helping feed information make all the difference

   a. Bad data in = bad data out; each department should be responsible for adequately and accurately communicating upcoming needs

   b. Best case/Worst case; in predictive modeling, we always want to include multiple scenarios. What is the best-case situation? What is the worst? Where is the middle ground and what is the likelihood of each occurring?

4. Look back and learn: This is a basic element of change management and one that definitely applies to rolling forecasts. Always look back to identify and document actual performance and data. This will inform your future predictions and forecasts.[16]

Saving Malpractice Expense

Medical malpractice coverage is a necessary and exorbitant expense for all providers. Though there are regulations at the state level (in some states) to help provide limit caps and endless lobbying from insurers, the fact remains that this will likely always be a large portion of your budget.

According to MarketWatch, "The global Medical Malpractice Insurance market size is projected to reach USD 17,410 million by 2027, from USD 14,560 million in 2020, at a CAGR of 2.6% during 2021-2027."[17] This really tells us that we can expect costs to continue to increase even though they vary widely by state. According to Statista, the top ten states with the highest medical malpractice premium expenses (respectively) are: New York, California, Pennsylvania, Florida, Illinois, New Jersey, Texas, Massachusetts, Maryland and Georgia.[18] If your organization is operating within any of these states, be sure to understand the legal medical malpractice environment to create risk-mitigation protocols based on claims trends.

There are ways to reduce medical malpractice premiums but they all require diligence:

1. Communicate

   a. Speak to your insurance broker and ask them for ways to obtain discounts. There may be safety training programs or other educational series for which participation can award a premium credit.

b. Talk to patients and be honest. It's been proven in several studies that strong relationships with physicians can reduce the likelihood of patient litigation. "One of the key factors [behind malpractice suits], appearing in 21% of our claims, is a lack of communication between the patient or their family and the physician."[19] The rapport your organization builds with your patient population could help minimize damages due to an adverse event.

c. Have an open-door policy for your workforce to bring concerns to your attention. Creating a culture of compliance will open the eyes and ears of everyone in your organization to be on the lookout for risk and report vulnerabilities.

2. Pay Ahead

a. When possible, pay your premiums in full. Premium costs are higher when the payments are split into quarterly or monthly invoices.

3. Consider a Deductible.

a. Deductibles can reduce malpractice premiums because it forces the provider or the practice to assume a portion of financial risk. "A deductible might shave 5% or 10% off of your annual insurance premium."[20]

4. Mitigate Risks

a. Employ the use of checklists, create patient safety guidelines and requirements for staff, educate staff on how to engage with upset patients.

b. The more you can mitigate risks to your malpractice insurance, the better chances you will minimize litigation and therefore minimize expense.

5. Audit Your Policy.

   a. Conduct an annual audit of your coverage, limits, and insureds. No one wants to find out that there are coverage gaps after a claim is made.

6. Slot Policy.

   a. Allows multiple part-time providers to essentially work as one full-time equivalent (FTE) provider based on the number of collective part-time hours equating to 1 FTE provider.

   b. There are significant cost savings as well as the flexible manner of reallocating hours for incoming providers to fill a slot left by an outgoing provider.

7. Participate in Hosted Activities

   a. Attend risk-based education programming offered by your medical malpractice carrier, when offered. Many of these programs will include continuing education units (CEUs) as well as credits that may be applied to your insurance premium for annual discounts.

   b. Encourage management and staff participation in education, surveys and other risk-mitigation activities hosted by your medical malpractice carrier to provide additional training and an overall culture of compliance education.

Remember, your liability carrier is your ally. To stay under the radar, many healthcare organizations steer clear of communicating much with their liability carrier out of fear of tripping the wire and letting on to potential internal risks. Throw that thinking in the trash and see them for what they are – on the same team. They have a vested interest in your claim reduction. Utilize them as a resource to discuss vulnerabilities and ask for risk mitigation advice. Rely on the education they provide to their policyholders on risk mitigation. You'll also find that they have best practice tools not only for the direct policy holders (i.e., physicians and non-physician practitioners (NPPs)), but also for ancillary and administrative office staff. Contact your malpractice carrier to determine what resources are available to your organization.

Public Contributions

In 2015, a study compared the US response to indigent care to that of other nations. The study found that "individual physician-based charity care obligations are unmanageable and unsuitable given the complexities of today's health care in the US."[21] Moreover, the article finds it unethical to assume that providers should take on the expense of indigent patients without support. It's a blunt opinion and there have been many comments on both sides of this argument. Whether you agree or disagree, the fact remains that charity care can be a significant burden to private practices.

Until different strategies are implemented nationwide, this is something that organizations need to implement individually. Here are some dos and don'ts for containing charity care expenses.

Do:

1. Require financial hardship applications
2. Evaluate applications based on the federal poverty level (FPL) and patient's ability to pay
3. Coordinate referral programs to transition patients who cannot afford care to state-funded, donation-funded, or non-profit facilities where applicable
4. Provide clear, written communication to patients about anticipated costs and their responsibilities
5. Utilize sliding fee schedules
6. Ask patients what they can afford to contribute

Do not:

- Offer blanket waivers of copays or deductibles
- Grant different discounts or charges without reason or structure

- Demean or threaten patients
- Refuse emergent care

1.6 Service and Site Variations – Costing, Evaluating, Reducing and Forecasting

Isn't it frustrating when you put in exhaustive effort toward planning, preparing and launching additional sites only to discover that for some reason they just aren't as profitable as other locations? Never mind the ever-annoying identification that the performance of a service is costing more for some providers than others. The challenge with variation is that it's almost never included in our initial plans. Our break-even analysis seldom includes the process erosion that often occurs in satellite offices or where service supply standards are not present. The best method to forecast the potential for variation is to first identify existing costs and evaluate the variance. From there, you can tackle reduction, and finally, projection into the future. The goal for all areas of evaluation is projection because that leads to process-perfecting and problem prevention.

Costing

In order to identify variance, you must be able to allocate costs appropriately. This means that expenses must be separated by location, allocated by service, or both.

Exhibit 1.11 Location Expense Comparison

Expense	Total	Location A	% Of Total	Location B	% Of Total
Medical Supplies	3,000,000	1,000,000	33.3%	2,000,000	66.7%
Provider Salaries	100,000,000	50,000,000	50%	50,000,000	50%
Facility Expenses	32,000	14,000	43.75%	18,000	56.25%
Total	**103,032,000**	**51,014,000**	**49.5%**	**52,018,000**	**50.5%**

This example isn't complex but it gives you the main idea. You want to review the same expense categories for each location, both individually and together, to ascertain the proportion they make up of the overall expense by category and by location. In the above example, the difference between the two sites is only 1%. At a glance, that number doesn't seem significant; however, the amount equates to over $1M. If we can achieve parity of expense by location, where Location B's expenses are reduced closer to that of Location A, any money saved reverts back to revenue for the organization.

In the above example, we see that the provider salaries are equivalent but the facility expense is much higher, as are the medical supplies. The variability of expenses for each facility location will also depend upon the location of each. If one location is in a metropolitan city, the facility, workforce and other expenses may vary based on an elevated cost of living. The site that is closest in proximity to the larger referral source (such as a hospital system) might receive a referral base that is larger in volume or service complexity. Another point of variation would be the types of testing and procedures available at each location. In the event that one location has been outfitted with specific medical equipment and technologists, that location may produce a higher net collection. Once we understand some of the challenges, we can look at the driving forces and refer back to the cost-containment section to help reduce variability between sites.

Again, the above is a very simplified version of what we want to see. Aim to include information that is pertinent to your organization. For example, you may want to include visit count, charges, adjustments, receipts, the prior year, etc. One format that is easy to use, yet informative, is reflected in the figure below, which you may recognize from MGMA's "Revenue Cycle Management: Don't Get Lost in the Financial Maze":

Exhibit 1.12 Sample Site Profitability Tool

Table 17.2 Sample Site Profitability Tool										
Annual Comparisons	Total Patient Visits		Charges		Adjustments		Net Collections		Expenses	
	Site 1	Site 2	Site 1	Site 2	Site 1	Site 2	Site 1	Site 2	Site 1	Site 2
Prior Year										
Trailing Year										
Year to Date										

Service Review and Forecasting

The purpose of a service variation review is to evaluate the cost differences by location and by provider. Imagine Dr. A and Dr. B perform the same services, but the supplies for Dr. A are twice the cost of Dr. B's. This difference provides insight into another area where cost can potentially be reduced. Likely you would want to review Dr. A's regular workflow against Dr. B's. Evaluate the difference in supplies used in terms of brand, cost, and quantity per service.

Your goal is to minimize variance to improve your ability to project future expenses for this service. Once you can do that, you can combine that information along with your fee schedule and historical service productivity numbers to project future profitability for performing this service. In addition, if the review identifies the service is being underpaid, then you can utilize the cost information as supporting evidence in contract negotiations.

Beyond the Concept

Once you have reduced operational costs and developed ongoing strategies for success, you should be able to make big operational changes comfortably, and these processes should give you the data and support required to validate or invalidate your decisions. Reduction of operational expense requires agile management, so you should be prepared to shift processes, vendors, or suppliers as needed. Mastery of this concept means you should:

1. Know what your costs are and why you have them (i.e., no surprises)

2. Have standardized products/supplies and have negotiated rates with vendors/suppliers with a strategy for sourcing high-demand items

3. Be prepared to optimize facility expenses, salaries and benefits, and insurance coverages

4. Be discerning about staff changes, facility design and technology use

5. Be always on the lookout for areas of opportunity, especially for high-cost categories

1.7 Case Study: Supply Savings

In 2018, RevCycle Intelligence published an article on healthcare supply chain costs which reviewed several pitfalls and successes as they relate to supply chain management.[22] One notable case referenced a health system in Georgia with 11 hospitals and over 200 additional locations.

The health system recognized rising supply costs in their surgical department and sought improvement by performing a product management and utilization oversight review with analysis by provider. The primary cause of their increased supply costs was identified as varied utilization of product and quantity by provider. In this situation, they could've mandated certain supplies and specifically allocated amounts. However, they decided to instead communicate the costs with providers and transparently share how they matched up against their peers' benchmark in terms of cost and utilization. By providing the actual data and associated context, the system realized double-digit savings for two separate procedures in just six weeks' time. Once their staff was "equipped with their own performance data, surgeons started to reduce supply chain costs on their own."[23]

There are two critical components of their success: evidence-based management and communication. Without access and review of their *actual* data, the organization would not have been able to present the challenges they were seeing with their costs. Similarly, merely having that information isn't enough. Driving real change requires staff engagement and participation. Sharing goals with your staff and pushing for team wins is a great way to achieve success while engaging staff as the company stakeholders they truly are. Cost containment with a side of corporate culture improvement? Why not!

Notes

1. https://www.investopedia.com/financial-edge/0711/the-cost-of-hiring-a-new
   -employee.aspx

2. https://www.paychex.com/articles/employee-benefits/twenty-low-cost-benefits-for-employees
3. https://www.hhs.gov/hipaa/for-professionals/privacy/guidance/access/index.html
4. https://www.cms.gov/newsroom/press-releases/cms-office-actuary-releases-2021-2030-projections-national-health-expenditures
5. https://www.ncbi.nlm.nih.gov/pmc/articles/PMC4450688/
6. https://hscrc.maryland.gov/Pages/tcocmodel.aspx#:~:text=To%20achieve%20a,other%20key%20demographics.%C2%A0%C2%A0
7. https://hscrc.maryland.gov/Pages/Statewide-Integrated-Health-Improvement-Strategy-.aspx
8. https://innovation.cms.gov/
9. https://revcycleintelligence.com/news/report-identifies-markets-ripe-for-payvider-adoption-growth
10. https://www.beckerspayer.com/payer/the-rise-of-the-payvider.html
11. https://www.beckershospitalreview.com/it-s-time-for-payvider-adoption-and-growth.html
12. https://www.banneraetna.com/en/about-us.html
13. https://guidehouse.com/-/media/www/site/insights/healthcare/2021/white-papers/now-is-the-time-for-payvider-adoption-growth.pdf
14. https://medcitynews.com/2021/06/report-which-us-markets-are-ripe-for-payvider-models/
15. https://www.healthcarefinancenews.com/news/dynamic-healthcare-budget-process-may-trump-traditional-budgeting-terms-accuracy-flexibility
16. https://www.afponline.org/ideas-inspiration/topics/articles/Details/8-steps-for-creating-a-rolling-forecast
17. https://www.marketwatch.com/press-release/medical-malpractice-insurance-market-2022-driving-factors-industry-growth-analysis-key-vendors-and-forecasts-to-2027-with-dominant-sectors-and-countries-data-2022-01-04
18. https://www.statista.com/statistics/796686/premiums-of-medical-professional-liability-insurance-usa-by-state/
19. https://www.medicaleconomics.com/view/how-avoid-malpractice-suits
20. https://www.physicianspractice.com/view/malpractice-insurance-how-lower-your-premiums
21. https://www.mdpi.com/2075-471X/4/2/201/pdf
22. https://revcycleintelligence.com/news/hospitals-could-save-25.4b-in-healthcare-supply-chain-costs
23. https://revcycleintelligence.com/features/data-analytics-add-value-to-healthcare-supply-chain-management

Chapter 2

Optimal Revenue Strategies

Defining and implementing optimal revenue strategies is more commonly referred to as "getting money in the door." This means providing valuable services, tackling bad debt, letting our data speak to us and support our planning efforts, and improving our rates of reimbursement. Let's face it, the absolute last thing we want to do is leave any portion of reimbursement uncollected, and we definitely don't want to miss out on opportunities to earn additional revenue. So how do we make sure we are optimizing our revenue strategies?

In order to optimize revenue strategies, we need to:

1. Provide value

2. Increase preventive care measures

3. Transition to value-based care and risk

4. Deal with bad debt

5. Use data and analytics as a financial predictor

6. Improve capture of patient A/R

7. Influence third-party payers

8. Create ancillary revenue streams

9. Evaluate and negotiate agreements carefully

2.1 Providing Value

The word "value" gets tossed around so often that it's almost starting to lose its own value; however, it's being mentioned for good reason. In order to optimize revenue, each organization must first confirm that the services being provided are worth reimbursing. Providing value in healthcare means more than providing a monetary equivalent of services, which is why the industry is moving away from fee-for-service (FFS) based models. So how do we define value now? According to the New England Journal of Medicine (NEJM), "Achieving high value for patients must become the overarching goal of health care delivery, with value defined as the health outcomes achieved per dollar spent."[1]

Providing value from the patient's perspective can look very different based on specialty, geographic region, and the patient's own goals. These differences are the reason why tying value to quantitative factors like outcomes and cost can be helpful in providing structure to value. That said, many have pointed out that focusing on costs and outcomes alone leaves the patient out of the value conversation. In order to create value for patients, ourselves, and the industry as a whole, we need to provide patients with communication, cost transparency, and top-notch customer service while evidencing to payers that there is genuine improvement in health outcomes and cost reduction.

Value-driven reimbursements have other benefits as well, "The pandemic exposed the shortcomings of fee-for-service while shining a light on the benefits of value-based contracts, which enabled organizations to pivot operations quickly and maintain revenue when volumes dropped."[2]

Measuring value from the payer's perspective will be similar across payer lines of business. At the heart of the matter, our payers judge our value to their ecosystem by our ability to provide them with healthcare cost-savings, accessibility to their beneficiaries, and successful outcomes. If your organization is falling behind on any of these metrics, then you are not demonstrating value to your payers and the result could impact your bottom line. In many markets, we are seeing payers terminate participation agreements and close their panels to high-cost, poor outcome providers.

Assessing Your Value

Determining your value can be challenging. Experts like Definitive Healthcare recommend focusing on these critical areas for analytics[3]:

1. Monitor the effectiveness of value-based care strategies

2. Identify opportunities to reduce cost across the organization

3. Improve clinical and quality scores through historical data tracking

Which key performance indicators (KPIs) you decide to use should be pertinent to your facility and services. If you don't refer patients for imaging services, then evaluating your MRI utilization or appropriate use criteria for imaging referrals wouldn't provide helpful information. Since we are focused on financial efforts for this book, consider the following KPIs as an example:

- Net Collections Ratio – of what was collectible, how much did you collect?
- Denial Rates – what percentage of claims are denied as the final determination?
- First Pass Denials – what percentage of claims are denied at first pass but eventually paid?
- Demographic Entry Accuracy – what is the percentage of data that is inaccurately entered by the front desk and intake staff?

2.2 Increasing Preventive Care Measures

Providing preventive care services adds a significant benefit to the patient care continuum. It can also be a positive force for your quality programs and revenue cycle overall. Most of us think of annual visits and vaccinations, but CMS actually includes many services under the preventive services list. A list of accepted preventive services includes:[4]

- Alcohol Misuse Screening & Counseling
- Annual Wellness Visits
- Bone Mass Measurements
- Cardiovascular Disease Screening Tests

- Cervical Cancer Screenings
- Colorectal Cancer Screenings
- Counseling to Prevent Tobacco Use
- Depression Screenings
- Diabetes Screenings
- Diabetes Self-Management Training (DMST)
- Flu Shot Administration
- Glaucoma Screenings
- Hepatitis B Screenings
- Hepatitis B Shot & Administration
- Hepatitis C Screenings
- HIV Screening
- IBT for Cardiovascular Disease
- IBT for Obesity
- Initial Preventive Physical Exam (IPPE)
- Lung Cancer Screenings
- Mammography Screenings
- Medical Nutrition Therapy (MNT)
- Medicare Diabetes Prevention Program (MDPP)
- Pap Screening Tests
- Pneumococcal Shot & Administration
- Prolonged Preventive Services
- Prostate Cancer Screenings
- STI Screening & HIBC to Prevent STIs
- Screening Pelvic Exams
- Ultrasound AAA Screenings
- *Note: CMS may update or revise this list at any time*

In addition to this list, CMS periodically adds additional preventive services. The push from CMS to include preventive services is evidence-based. According to the Office of Disease Prevention and Health Promotion, "Getting preventive care reduces the risk for diseases, disabilities, and death — yet millions of people in the United States don't get recommended preventive health care services."[5] When diseases, disabilities, and deaths are not prevented, there is higher expense to the industry overall.

Preventive Services Revenue

Not all specialties can provide preventive services, but those that can should evaluate the potential benefits to patient care and facility revenue that can occur. For example, a practice with 5,000 existing Medicare beneficiaries that reaches an 85% performance rate on

Annual Wellness Visits (AWV) at the 2022 National CMS payment rate of $132.54 would receive an additional $563k in revenue from that one service alone. If they can increase the performance rates or if any of the patients are receiving their first ever AWV, that amount increases. Though CMS doesn't have a reportable clinical quality measure (CQM) for AWVs, many commercial carriers do. For example, Highmark's Medicare Advantage plan has CQM C51 included on their list of required performance measures for 2022.[6]

Integrating Preventive Services Protocols

The implementation or integration of technologies can be stressful for providers and staff, but the benefits of having technology to support new initiatives can outweigh that burden. This is also true for the integration and optimization of preventive services. To integrate a full-scale preventive services program successfully:

1. Evaluate the services that fit your practice and align with the needs of your patient community.

2. Develop a preventive services tracker in your EHR system by creating a checklist of the applicable services. Many systems already have a method for this or track it automatically through billed services.

3. Make sure that the checklist allows for the services to be checked off as well as dated. This is important as there are typically strict timelines for how often preventive services can be billed.

4. Run regular reports to identify the services that are not being performed and evaluate why those opportunities were missed.

5. Develop a culture of continuous process optimization so that preventive service performance increases over time.

6. Provide preventive service education to patients online, on social media, in pamphlets, and in the exam room.

When it comes to implementing preventive service programs and establishing a regular cadence with patients, it's important to keep in mind that you do not have to reinvent the wheel. A lot of research has been done at the state, federal, and even global level on best practice prevention programs. For example, SAMHSA has guidance for practitioners who want to establish substance misuse prevention programs,[7] *JAMA* has been publishing evidence-based research on preventive service programs for decades, and Veterans Affairs has a step-by-step guide for program implementation at their facilities which they made available for public use.[8] An effectively run value-based program can result in healthier patients, increased revenue, and more successful value-based program scores.

With the expansion of price transparency, high-deductible plans, No Surprises Act, value-based care, and Pay for Performance, our consumers are savvy and have choices. Just as they shop on Amazon and other consumer-driven service platforms, healthcare organizations need to adapt to patients' needs to manage the costs of their own care. Patients are more interested in determining their total cost of care as they leverage health savings accounts, flexible spending accounts, and other healthcare-spending solutions. Patients will no longer rely solely on a practitioner's reputation to make decisions related to care – they are informed consumers and require good faith estimates, payment plans, credit cards kept on file for future care, and estimates of coinsurance amounts.

Collectively, healthcare providers should lead patients in financial literacy, illness/injury prevention, linkage to medical care, and adherence to treatment plans to reduce out-of-pocket healthcare expenses. To increase utilization of the patient-centered medical home concept and reduce emergency room visits, healthcare practitioners should improve patient education and resources for owning the management of one's own healthcare.

The entire healthcare system wins when patients are educated on navigating these complex healthcare systems so that they reduce acute and chronic onset of illnesses, which improves outcomes and satisfaction while reducing overall healthcare costs. We have a unique opportunity to optimize patients' use of technology in the management of their own care to strengthen current collaborative care through patient portals, remote patient monitoring and telehealth services. Patients who are at risk for increasing healthcare spending are those with Social Determinants of Health (SDOH). According to the U.S. Department of Health and Human Services, "Social determinants of health are the conditions in the environments where people are born, live, learn, work, play, worship, and age that affect a wide range of health functioning and quality-of-life outcomes and risks.[9]" An educated patient is armed to make informed medical decisions. It's not enough to have practitioners working on managing costs – we must engage our patients in these efforts in order to truly succeed.

2.3 Transitions to VBP and Risk

Health plans, Accountable Care Organizations (ACOs), and other entities that utilize a risk-based approach to payments use this data to predict healthcare costs for a population. These predictions are then used to forecast payment to providers or offer distributions for shared savings for rendering services to a population. You may be asking yourself what happens when payment calculations are inaccurate. Glad you asked. When risk-based payment forecasts are inaccurate, payments and shared savings distributions are not calculated correctly. Again, you may be asking yourself why these forecasts would be inaccurate. One way that these forecasts could be inaccurate is based on the data received in provider documentation. Accurate depiction and description of illnesses is key. When an illness is listed as unspecified, it lacks the detail and level of complexity needed by health plans, ACOs and other entities that use illness-related data to make predictions on total cost of care.

Ultimately, Total Cost of Care refers to the total cost of providing healthcare for a population. In order to determine total cost of care, one needs to identify costs associated with care delivery. Reducing and managing total cost of care requires collaboration, transformation, and shared financial risk. Throughout this section we will examine each of these components.

Collaborative Service Arrangements

Accountable Care Organizations (ACOs) and Clinically Integrated Networks (CINs) are formed for and are sustainable with the goal of cost containment for savings distributions. As the overhaul of healthcare was underway through the ACA legislation, the ACO model was birthed by CMS to hold these entities accountable for cost reduction and quality improvement for the Medicare beneficiaries within their panel. In order for ACOs to be successful, their organization must provide collaborative rather than siloed care within its network of providers.

Now that it's been proven that ACOs can increase revenue by taking on risk, there has been significant growth in the ACO model. Factors that ACOs take into consideration when measuring risk vs reward are their ability to prevent unnecessary hospitalizations as well as prevent readmissions by aligning hospital system resources with community physicians under one ACO. Under the ACO model, providers are now on the hook for financial accountability for total cost of care which incentivizes provider shifts in decision making for items such as test ordering, use of drug formularies, and clinical decision support (CDS) programmed within an EMR.

The ACO payment structure includes fee-for-service payments during the performance year as well as payment adjustments based on success of quality performance, which results in either a Medicare Shared Savings Program (MSSP) payment distribution or penalty. The MSSP payment distribution is calculated based on the savings that the ACO accumulated throughout the performance period. This payment is also based on the agreed upon performance metrics and the success rate of each. When entering into risk-based contracts, it's critical to ensure close monitoring of provider performance, habits, and compliance, as these elements will surely impact the entire group either negatively or positively based on the provider's ability to adhere to pre-established guidelines.

Exhibit 2.1 Shared Savings Program Map[10]

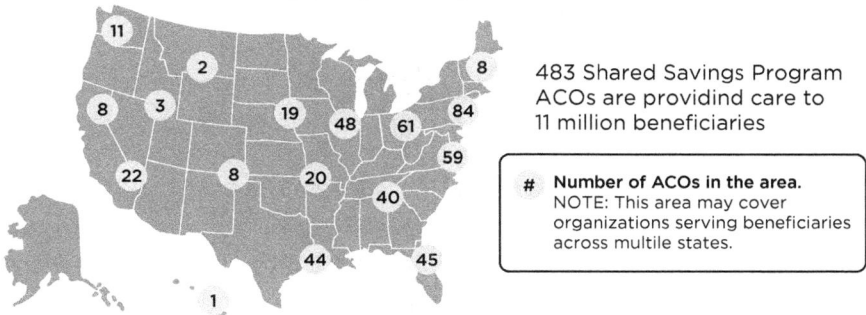

483 Shared Savings Program ACOs are providind care to 11 million beneficiaries

**Number of ACOs in the area.**
NOTE: This area may cover organizations serving beneficiaries across multile states.

Many organizations, including ACOs, may participate in more than one value-based program. Measuring success in a cross-functional manner creates a birds-eye view of all programs and measures as well as the success of each. It is then much easier to apply the same Clinical Quality Measures (CQMs) that are being tracked across programs.

Exhibit 2.2 Sample CQM Matrix

Program	MIPS	PCMH	HEDIS	EPSDT	APM
Diabetes eye exam	X	X	X		
Diabetic Foot Exam	X	X	X		
A1C	X	X	X		
Blood Pressure Control	X	X	X		X
Lung Cancer reporting	X				
Preventive care and screening: BMI and follow up plan	X	X	X	X	X
Influenza vaccine	X	X	X	possible	
Radiology Dose Exposure or Time Reported for procedures using fluoroscopy	X				
Reminder system for screening mammograms	X	X			
Labs	X	X	X	X	X
Colorectal Cancer Screening	X	X			
Physical Exam			X	X	X
Heart Failure Beta Blocker for LVSD	X	X			X

51

Program	MIPS	PCMH	HEDIS	EPSDT	APM
Hypertension: Improvement in Blood Pressure	X	X			
Depression screening	X	X	X	X	X

In the above example, the facility has sorted the programs they participate in alongside services which apply to multiple programs. As you can see, there are multiple services that impact every program the facility participates in, which gives them insight for prioritizing their focus on CQMs for the largest impact. Having a CQM matrix kills multiple birds with one stone. Since many measures overlap in multiple programs, one can track each measure across programs.

The CMS aims to reach 100% of its original Medicare beneficiaries and the majority of Medicaid beneficiaries with some form of value-based care by 2030. One of these models that has grown in popularity is the formation of Clinically-Integrated Networks (CINs). Similar to the ACO model, there are many benefits to CINs: better control of medical expenses, robust clinical outcomes, and pricing stability. CINs also enable participants to collaborate on care, creating better financial relationships between CIN participants. However, you do need to be wary of forming a CIN. One of the most common struggles organizations face is utilizing different EHR systems. Providers need to be able to share data across the organization to be as efficient as possible. Physicians entering a CIN must be willing to provide the resources required to effectively manage their total cost of care.[11]

Value-based program participation requires a ton of coordination and workflow efficiencies for promoting interoperability, practice improvement activities, quality measures, and overall cost improvements. Each of these requirements is included in daily revenue cycle workflows and can be mapped to revenue cycle components to identify, modify, and improve outcomes.

Utilize the revenue cycle to map workflows as seen in the image on the next page.

Exhibit 2.3 Value-Based Workflow Mapping

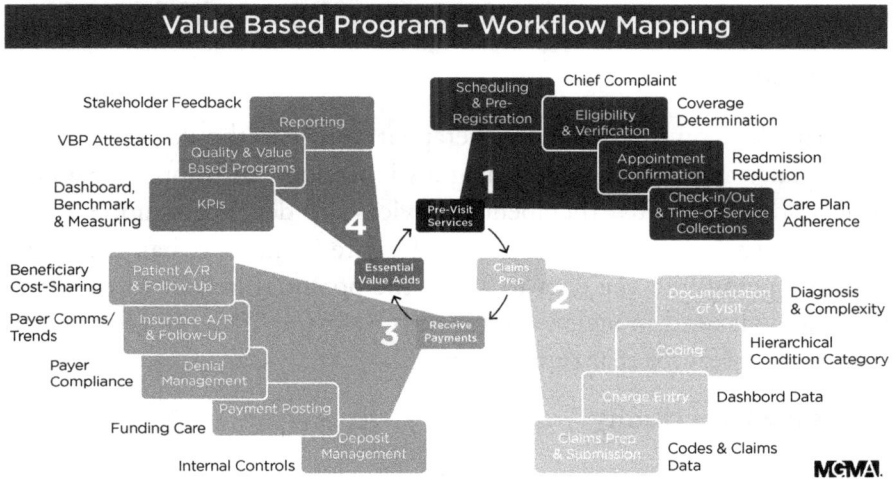

2.4 Creating Revenue Streams

Diversifying revenue streams can be essential for the long-term success of the organization. The challenge is creating something of value to the community as well as the facility while also ensuring the task isn't too large to take on. "Most physician practices — 82% — offer at least one ancillary service."[12]

The two main types of ancillary services an organization can provide, in addition to the primary service offering, are diagnostic and therapeutic.

Diagnostic Services

Implementing diagnostic services can be a significant benefit depending on how services are implemented. The largest benefit after revenue for diagnostic services is the control associated with testing. With in-house testing, the facility is able to perform the testing and read the results much sooner than through patient referrals to external facilities. The most frequently implemented diagnostic services are laboratory testing, radiology/imaging services, and specialty-specific services (like cardiac monitoring, audiology, etc.); "84% of family medicine and 73% of internal medicine practices offer electrocardiography."[13]

Therapeutic Services

The decision to implement therapeutic services should be evaluated by specialty and scope. Where diagnostic testing can inform a patient's conditions and status, therapeutic services are dependent upon medical necessity. So, one is necessary much more frequently than the other. Before digging into the data to assess the potential benefit to the practice, you will need to review your facility's existing data on referrals and treatment orders for that type of service.

Assess the Opportunity

Implementing ancillary services really equates to looking for additional revenue opportunities. Decisions to move forward should be given the same amount of scrutiny as other investment opportunities and should consider the following:

1. Evaluate the cost of implementation as well as the fixed and variable costs per rendered service
    a. Facility
        i. Will you need to expand?
        ii. Does the service require construction (example: lead-lined walls for radiology machines)?
    b. Machine and service contract expenses
    c. Software, computers, printers, and integration expenses
    d. Training/education
    e. Additional staff
    f. Licenses/certifications
    g. Inspection fees
    h. Insurance coverage
        i. Will you need changes to malpractice, general liability, or workers' compensation policies in order to provide this service?

    i. Professional fees

        i. Legal opinion

        ii. Consultant

        iii. Other professional services

2. Identify revenue opportunities

    a. Are services covered under existing payer agreements or will negotiations be required?

    b. Are services covered by most insurers? Do they often require prior authorizations? Will you need to obtain an advanced beneficiary notification (ABN) for services?

    c. In what situations is the service considered medically necessary and how frequently does that occur?

3. Calculate the best-case, worst-case, and most-likely productivity scenarios

    a. Estimate the time to break-even on each

4. Review community demographics/ market readiness

5. Identify competition and impact to projected service utilization

6. Discuss with attorney or compliance advisors

    a. Ensure there are no conflicts with STARK Law

    b. Is the service within the scope of practice for the facility and providers?

    c. Are there federal, state, or regional restrictions to providing this service?

2.5 Contract Evaluation and Negotiation

Insurance reimbursement is the largest revenue source for most healthcare organizations. According to Kaiser Family Foundation (KFF), "Most non-pediatric office-based physicians accept new Medicare patients (89%), as well as new private insurance patients (91%)."[14] This statistic requires us to place high importance on how we engage insurance companies when entering into legally binding participation agreements. Insurance companies rely on contract language that provides favorable terms and conditions for them, but what about healthcare organizations?

The authors would like to thank Kevin Mulcahy, FACMPE, senior director of provider and payer service, Mass General Physician Organization, who collaborated with us on this topic.

Understanding Your Market

As we seek to engage with payers, we must live in their world by continually staying abreast of their regional footprint and overall impact to the organization and patient populations. To truly get a lay of the land, we must identify the local and national payers – as well as the predominant Medicaid MCOs: commercial payers. It's also wise to identify workers' compensation, motor vehicle and international funding sources – segregation of these payer mixes from others is key as we assure rates are at or above commercial levels. Yes, not only must we research these entities, we should also be able to answer these critical questions about each:

1. What is the targeted payer's position in the marketplace? Have they recently been acquired, merged or been considering similar transactions?

2. How many leadership changes have occurred with the targeted payer in the last 24 months?

3. What is the targeted payer's long-term viability, growth expectations and product expansion plan for the next 2-3 years?

4. What is my organization's value in the marketplace?

5. What differentiates your organization from other healthcare provider organizations?

6. Who is responsible for payer contracting for your organization? (practice administrator, IPA, CIN, ACO, MSO, health system)

○ Who is the voice of your contracting table?

○ What communication process is used to ultimately accept or reject a contract?

The first three questions, once answered, assist with determining the strengths and weaknesses of the targeted payer as you develop your negotiation strategy. Leadership changes may signify instability or growth which you should plan to solve for in your value proposition.

Each market is different. The Midwest market may differ from the East Coast. Recognize that each market will vary and focus on differentiating your organization. By thoughtfully answering questions four and five above, you can demonstrate why a payer should keep your organization in-network. Then seek to negotiate terms that fit your needs for participation.

Question number six is an important consideration when your organization is not negotiating on its own behalf. In these cases, the healthcare organization would delegate this responsibility to one person or one entity and refer all matters of negotiation to that person/entity to assure continuity and alignment. This is typically through a binding authority process. Binding authority is when each person, "signing the agreement on behalf of either party individually warrants that he or she has full legal power to execute this agreement on behalf of the party for whom he or she is signing, and to bind and obligate such party with respect to all provisions contained in the agreement."[15]

Evaluating Actual Payments Against Expected Negotiated Payments

A critical component of a payer participation agreement is the fee schedule. The fee schedule is an outline of CPT/HCPCS, DME, supplies, and other reimbursable items by a health plan or funding source. The payment rate or allowed amount for each item is included in the fee schedule. The allowed amount is unique to each payer – many of which use Medicare's rates as a benchmark to reimburse for medical services. Payers use payment formulas that take into consideration some of the following factors:

1. Utilization review

2. Usual and customary / Geographic area pricing

3. Relative value units (Work and practice RVUs)

4. Cost

5. Outcomes

6. Medicare's conversion factor

7. National coverage determination (NCD) and local coverage determination (LCD) policies

This is where we roll up our sleeves to determine whether or not we're getting paid what we are owed – according to our contracted rates. As many of us are relying on electronic payment posting, there are opportunities to track and trend payment posting by uploading your organization's payer fee schedules to your practice management software to receive under- or overpayment alerts. Create posting rules for billing staff based upon contract terms and allowable rates to support the identification of payment variances. There's also the manual process of developing a spreadsheet and plugging in data from remittance advice to identify trends.

One must know a payer's reimbursement rules as they pertain to multiple services provided on the same date of service, as well as the reimbursement or impact of a procedure performed on the same date of service as an E&M code. Most will require a modifier, but again, these rules are important to understand and follow in order to ensure you're comparing apples to apples.

Organizations that rely significantly on E&M codes or other small code sets may find themselves diverting to a manual fee schedule review, while larger or multispeciality organizations may need to use software for review.

Payer Contract Evaluation Work Plan Process

- Articulate the basis of your organization's interest in participating with:
  - A new payer, potential contract, or product line
  - New employer-sponsored health insurance coverage for existing patients

- ○ New product offering by payer
- ○ Medicare Advantage or Medicaid Managed Care
- Develop objectives and appetite for potential contract
- Identify your cost to charge ratio so that you may develop a target reimbursement rate that the practice is willing to accept
- Determine your reimbursement pricing flexibility
- Identify risk-sharing criteria and the financial implications both positively and negatively
- Understand and be included in the selection of data being used to evaluate the financial risk
- Clearly determine obligations for quality reporting

As part of the contract evaluation work plan, it's also wise to identify non-rate factors that impact the cost of doing business in order to achieve administrative simplification with the goal of reducing practice expenses. Explore No Referral opportunities to cut down on uncompensated workflows that add little to no value to your organization or patients. Determining carve-out for prior authorizations and referrals and replacing them with referral within a local network that shares clinical data systems should be done to minimize the referral process. This process also reduces administrative expenses and provides seamless care for the patient. Ensure payers can accept HIPAA-compliant transactions to eliminate paper billing and appeals processes. This should include the acceptance of attachments electronically, including but not limited to notes, other payer information for coordination of benefits (COB), electronic remittance advice (ERA), and electronic funds transfers (EFTs).

Successfully Negotiating Payer Contracts

We may elevate our income potential by expanding our knowledge on payer reimbursement models so that we can optimize our fee schedules and payer contract language and terms. It's true that many payers' contract language is boilerplate and based on some nationally recognized law firm's due diligence on behalf of said payer. Our focus when analyzing our payer participation agreements should be the opportunity to add services not mentioned in the agreement, remove or carve out language and terms that we find overly burdensome or inappropriate for our specialty or region, and negotiate our fee schedules. Yes, you heard that right. *Negotiate your payments in advance.* Many of us have already entered into payer participation agreements but it's not too late to do a full payer contract analysis and fee schedule negotiation.

There is a playbook to contract and fee schedule negotiations so that both parties win. It's all about getting to the yes; in order for any negotiation to work, both parties (providers and health plans) need to be willing to compromise and successfully walk away from the experience of having gained something they determine is worthwhile. So, what does a win look like for each party? The healthcare provider is expecting higher reimbursement and hopefully a reduction in administrative burdens (i.e., pre-authorizations, timely filing limits). The health plan may feel that they have won if the internal cost structure is not compromised by increasing rates and they are able to keep the most highly skilled low-cost providers in-network.

Many healthcare provider organizations skip contract and fee schedule negotiations altogether out of concern that the behemoth insurance company would never consider changing a word in their contracts, let alone increasing the reimbursement. It's true, there are times that health plans will decline negotiation requests. The health plan may respond with an outright no that lacks any rationale for their decision. How do you get around this? Again, glad you asked. Use a tactic offered by Roger Fisher and William Ury known as, "Negotiation Jujitsu."[16] If they won't play ball, pull their attention from your initial request and move it toward the merits of your request. Take the focus away from the ask and highlight the merits.

There are three methods to focus the negotiation discussion on merits. Before you deploy these methods, get your data and ducks in a row. Use these three "Negotiation Jujitsu" tactics to get them to focus on merits rather than a request. Demonstrate:

1. What you can do – Can you lower their expenditures? Can you keep their beneficiaries out of the hospital? Can you better manage chronic illnesses? Can you keep their beneficiaries happy through excellent customer service? Can you demonstrate illness complexity and medical

necessity through medical documentation? Can their beneficiaries reach you when they need you?

Exhibit 2.4 HEDIS Domains[17]

Each rated health plan has an overall quality rating of 1 to 5 stars (5 is highest), The 6 HEDIS domains include: Effectiveness of Care, Access/ Availability of Care, Experience of Care, Utilization and Risk Adjusted Utilization, Health Plan Descriptive Information and Measures Reported Using Electronic Clinical Data Systems. -www.ncqa.org/hedis

2. What they can do – They can boost their star rating by keeping your provider in-network as your provider is offering optimal medical care which bolsters their rating. They can improve their HEDIS performance and measurements (member experience, medical care and health plan administration) by keeping your provider in-network while having a policy of increasing office hours – which may expand provider availability as well as demonstrate effectiveness of care based on medical record documentation offered by your organization. Both are HEDIS measures by which health plans are measured based on effectiveness. They can avoid patients having to change providers by keeping your organization in-network. They can reduce readmissions and hospital-acquired infections by having in-network providers who offer telehealth services, have after-hours, before-hours, and weekend appointment options.

Exhibit 2.5 HEDIS Definition[18]

Healthcare Effectiveness Data and Information Set (HEDIS) is a comprehensive set of standardized performance measures designed to provide purchasers and consumers with the information they need for reliable comparison of health plan performance. -www.cms.gov

3. What a third party (patient) can do – That's right guys; we're pulling out the big guns here. The patient is the consumer for both parties – and the healthcare provider has a care delivery relationship with this "third party." This third party (patient) has leverage over the providers and health insurance they choose. Granted, some patients are limited in their health plan selection based on options made available by their employers. Health plans should not, however, under-estimate the power of the provider-patient relation-ship. Many patients will follow their provider to the ends of the earth if they've built a strong relationship based on mutual trust, illness management, and bed-side manner.

Now that we've gotten the health plan to play ball, we can focus on getting both parties to an agreement that's a win-win for everyone. Let's start our negotiation strategy to improve our income by analyzing our contract language. Remember, once executed, these are legally binding terms. Make sure you review these documents carefully. Below is a list of routine contract terms to become familiar with as you manage the contract evaluation and negotiation process.

Exhibit 2.6 Routine Payer Contract Language

Payer Participation Language	Analysis	Income Consideration
Agreement Type	Indicates whether the contract is a group contract or a solo-provider contract. In the event you have multiple providers in your practice, you'll want a group contract.	There will be billing limitations on a solo-provider contract. There will also be the lack of economies of scale for a solo-provider contract.
Product Selections	Itemization of the payer products your organization agrees to accept assignment.	Opt out of products with low reimbursement or complex administrative functions that will increase overhead thereby decreasing reimbursement.

Payer Participation Language	Analysis	Income Consideration
Electronic Data Interchange (EDI) Number	Should be entered into the organization's practice management and/or clearinghouse.	Required for electronic claim submission. 10–14-day payment turnaround.
Provider Directory	Ensure that there's mention about accessing the online provider directory and the health plan's responsibility to keep it up to date.	Inaccurate records will be a barrier to patient's accessing your providers – decreasing your patient volumes.
Contract Term	Many contracts will have an automatic renewal. Determine the termination notice requirements.	Might be used as leverage during contract and fee schedule negotiations.
Timely Claims Submission	Ensure these guidelines follow your state's rules. Some payers use the TFL rules for the state of their corporate headquarters.	A decreased timely filing limit will create a financial burden in the event your practice needs extra time to submit claims.
Clean Claim Payment	Ensure these guidelines follow your state's rules. Some payers use the TFL rules for the state of their corporate headquarters.	An increased claim payment timeline will delay payments being received by your organization.
Termination for Breach	Stuff happens. Rogue providers and other factors may cause a breach. Identify them, and update employment contracts and employee manuals to avoid breaches from occurring.	Breaches will be costly. Manage them accordingly. Prepare your organization for the consequences by being proactive. Calculate financial fall-out.
Amendments	Many contract amendments are deemed as automatically accepted if there is no response.	Amendments may include decreased reimbursement so be sure that they are always reviewed. Respond in the timeframe listed if you do not agree.
Correspondence, Service, Pay to Address	The addresses listed on the contract are the addresses that will be used by the health plan. Ensure the complete accuracy of this information and send changes on practice letterhead – certified, return receipt.	Payments might be sent to the wrong location if information is not accurate. Claims may be denied if the service address is incorrect.

Payer Participation Language	Analysis	Income Consideration
Group / Provider Roster	This should be an accurate listing of all providers you would like to be included in the participation agreement.	Missing providers will be excluded from reimbursement. Other claims processing issues may occur.
State Compliance Addendum	Ensure the health plan is using the state in which services will be provided if the addendum is included.	Contact your state's insurance commissioner if your state's compliance guidelines are not being used.
Medical Rental Product Participation	Transfer or subcontracting of provider participation with the provider's written consent.	Most MRNs or Third Parties will utilize their own plan payment terms which you have no access to review or agree.
Fee Schedule	Usual and customary rates for services performed based on specialty and geographic location. Sometimes a "sample" fee schedule will be provided – which should be refused.	Ensure the fee schedule is assigned to your organization. Review fee schedule to ensure all CPT/HCPCS for your organization are listed. Negotiate rates of reimbursement.

Ideally, you'll want to have an executive summary for each payer participation agreement that includes a matrix indicating the effective date, termination/expiration date, and months that are open for negotiations.

Yes, that's right – many contracts allot negotiation windows, so be sure to know yours. These windows could be a timeframe selected by the payer such as the second quarter of the year. It could be 3–6 months prior to the contract expiration date. Negotiating contract language may help improve your income by identifying administratively burdensome tasks like being required to obtain pre-authorization for routine services. Calculate the manpower it takes, the frequency, and the revenue lost to formulate your income increase after having carved out this process.

Answer these questions:

1. Does the product offering of the contract complement your practice?

   a. Does it bring new lines of business that you are willing to accept?

   b. Identifying the types of patients the payer covers and who exactly in your practice is responsible for managing a patient's care is imperative. Most payers offer an array of products from traditional commercial employer-sponsored plans to government-sponsored Medicare and Medicaid replacement plans. A practice must understand the payer's overall product offerings and covered lives within products.

2. What is the payer's distribution of membership within these products? This helps with understanding the patient population covered within the contract.

3. Within the products they are offering in your marketplace do they have:

   a. Network limitations? – This may impede access to the highest level of benefits to the patient; unknowingly increasing a patient's out-of-pocket financial responsibility.

     i. Are all provider types (e.g., NP, PA) eligible to participate in all products?

     ii. Will referral patterns be required to shift for inpatient/outpatient, lab, radiology and surgical services or is your practice aligned appropriately with participating providers?

4. Tiering? – Increased patient liability due to copays and coinsurance based upon the tiering level of your practice or individual provider. Understand what is required to improve a provider's assigned tier.

5. Opt-out capabilities? – Do providers have the ability to individually opt out of participation with certain plans?

6. What entity is actually responsible for payment of claims?

   a. Understanding the percentage of the payers' beneficiaries who are fully insured patients and self-insured members is key. Fully insured members' payments are the responsibility of the payer. For self-insured members, while the payment is transmitted via the payer, the payment is ultimately the responsibility of the employer. Payers or networks that represent self-insured employers are only a network that provide claims administration and a network of providers. Therefore, if the employer does not fund the payment of claims, payment will be delayed to the practice. Differentiating a fully insured member from a self-insured patient is not easy and payers do not typically disclose that information at the patient level.

7. Does the network provide you with appropriate referral support should you need to refer the patient to another provider or facility?

8. What type of payment method is utilized for reimbursement?

   a. Fee for Service

   b. Pay for Performance

   c. Shared Risk

   d. Capitated or Bundled

Organizational Value of Payer Contract Management

There is little incentive for attorneys working on behalf of insurance companies to include overly favorable terms on behalf of healthcare organizations. A comprehensive understanding of payer participation agreements and best practices for ensuring favorable contract terms and reimbursement rates is necessary when optimizing income opportunities in the healthcare setting. Doing so will provide healthcare organizations with the ability to formulate favorable participation and service reimbursement terms.

With so many reimbursement methodologies to keep track of, follow, and optimize, healthcare organizations that prioritize payer contract management see greater reimbursement results. Once a contract has been established, there are key drivers for implementing and overseeing a contract management system. Several drivers include when, why, and how often your organization is being paid different amounts for the same CPT/ HCPCS codes, identifying as well as resolving under- and overpayments for revenue integrity, and adhering to payers' reimbursement guidelines such as bundling rules. There are costs associated with payer participation, so understanding your costs to play is critical to successful participation.

Areas to consider for internal assessment include:

- Determine if your practice management system (PMS) has a contract management module
- Understand and agree to key terms, conditions and contract language
- Consider how your organization's particular specialty of services is paid along with the complexity of payment rules for your specialty (e.g., Primary Care or specialty-based organization with complex services that may require testing or procedures)
- Percentage of Evaluation and Management services performed
- Payer Mix
- Products/lines of business included in the contract
- Determination whether Third-Party Administrators (TPAs) manage claim payments or if contracts can be outsourced to medical rental networks
- Does your practice management system have financial categories by payer?
- Can you identify your commercial patients from your Medicare Advantage patients that are covered by the same payer?
- Identify individuals within your organization who are responsible and accountable for reviewing and communicating payer policy changes, reimbursement changes, and reacting. This can be someone in your billing over-the-counter Cash Management

We can move in the direction of success at the outset by being prepared for negotiations and identifying the terms, conditions and rates that are suitable for our organizations. Utilize your payer participation agreements as an opportunity to increase income.

Beyond the Concept

Demonstrating value to a payer may include the development, management, and distribution of a value proposition. The value proposition explains to payers the benefits of having your group empaneled and in-network. Payers rely on their in-network providers to improve or maintain their internal quality or star ratings. Health plan star ratings are based on:[19]

1. Member experience – Based on satisfaction surveys with their healthcare and doctors, ease of obtaining appointments and services.

2. Medical care – Based on the way network providers manage the members' healthcare such as regular screenings, vaccines, basic services and monitoring patients' conditions.

3. Plan administration – Based on how well the health plan is being run to include levels of customer service, access to information, and in-network providers who order appropriate tests and treatment.

Components of an effective value proposition include value-based program scoring of Merit-Based Incentive Payment System (MIPS) program measures, Healthcare Effectiveness Data and Information Set (HEDIS) measures, internal patient satisfaction survey results, avoidance of emergency rooms and unnecessary hospitalizations, readmission prevention through transitional care management programs and hospital collaborations, integrated care models such as Accountable Care Organization (ACO), Clinically Integrated Network (CIN) and Independent Physician Association (IPA) participation. Additional factors to be included in a value proposition would be organizational process improvement strategies, appointment availability before and after typical business hours, industry recognitions and certifications, location in an underserved or shortage area and offering of in-demand specialty services.

Utilize the below questionnaire to extract key metrics that demonstrate your organization's success in Value-Based Program participation for inclusion in your value proposition.

Exhibit 2.7 Value Proposition Questionnaire

Total number of providers by specialty	
Practice specialties	
Total number of active patients	
Do you provide 24/7 coverage?	
Do you have an active patient portal?	
Do providers have real-time EMR access outside of the facility?	
What are your 2-year value-based programs' scores by reporting year and program?	
How do you track continuity of care?	
How quickly can patients get access to care?	
Do you provide telehealth services?	
What is your organization's process / philosophy on case management?	
How do you track patient emergency department (ED) or hospital discharges?	
What steps do you follow for comprehensive medication management?	
How do you coordinate referral management for specialists and/or primary care services?	

Exhibit 2.8 Access to Care and Communications

Services	Never	Rarely	Sometimes	Often	Always
Same- or next-day appointments					
Telephone advice during office hrs.					
Virtual or telephone advice during weekends					

Services	Never	Rarely	Sometimes	Often	Always
Virtual or telephone advice after hours					
Secure/encrypted email / pt portal					
Wait time to schedule urgent/acute appointments?					
Wait time to schedule routine follow-up visits?					
Wait time to schedule chronic disease management visit?					
Wait time to schedule physical exam if applicable?					
Wait time to schedule Annual Wellness Visit (AWV) if applicable?					

Table: Value Proposition Questionnaire Using Value-Based Program Participation Data

2.7 Case Study

In 2019, a solo dermatologist on the East Coast was seeing an increase in volume from Payer 1. This payer represented 60% of the dermatologist's payer mix; however, this payer was the second-lowest payer on this physician's roster. Payer 1 also required a significant number of prior-authorizations and referrals for dermatologic services, thereby creating a higher administrative output, which required the hiring of additional staff. Upon completion of a fee schedule analysis, payer participation agreement review, and staff allocation analysis, it was determined that participation with Payer 1 was no longer profitable for the physician.

A market analysis confirmed that the physician was located in a geographic region that was properly supported by the payer. However, the dermatologist specialized in a specific service that others did not – making the dermatologist's in-network affiliation beneficial to the payer and its members. The dermatologist purchased necessary equipment that allowed for this specialized service to be performed in the office in an out-patient setting rather than at an Ambulatory Surgical Center (ASC) or hospital – saving the health plan on facility fees and other related expenses.

Through a value proposition and effective negotiations, the dermatologist was able to successfully create prior-authorization carve-outs within the participation agreement so that certain services would be exempt from referral or prior-authorization requirements – thereby decreasing the physician's administrative burden which allowed staff to focus those efforts on patient care. Payer 1 also increased seven CPT codes by 15% along with an overall rate increase from 100% of Medicare to 150% of Medicare. The Dermatologist is still in-network with Payer 1.

Notes

1. https://www.nejm.org/doi/full/10.1056/nejmp1011024

2. https://revcycleintelligence.com/features/value-based-contracting-101-preparing-negotiating-and-succeeding

3. https://www.definitivehc.com/blog/success-in-value-based-care

4. https://www.cms.gov/Medicare/Prevention/PrevntionGenInfo/medicare-preventive-services/MPS-QuickReferenceChart-1.html

5. https://health.gov/

6. https://content.highmarkprc.com/Files/Region/navinet/ValueBasedProg/MAStars/2022-MAIP.pdf

7. https://www.samhsa.gov/

8. https://www.prevention.va.gov/prevention_leader_resources/stepbystepmanual.pdf

9. https://health.gov/healthypeople/objectives-and-data/social-determinants-health

10. https://www.cms.gov/Medicare/Medicare-Fee-for-Service-Payment/ACO

11. https://www.cms.gov/blog/cms-innovation-centers-strategy-support-person-centered-value-based-specialty-care

12. https://www.beckersasc.com/asc-coding-billing-and-collections/how-much-revenue-do-ancillary-services-generate-3-survey-insights.html?oly_enc_id=3214E4523789H7B

13. https://payrhealth.com/resources/blog/expand-your-practice-with-ancillary-care-services/

14. https://www.kff.org/medicare/issue-brief/most-office-based-physicians-accept-new-patients-including-patients-with-medicare-and-private-insurance/

15. https://www.lawinsider.com/clause/binding-on-physicians

16. https://www.pon.harvard.edu/daily/negotiation-skills-daily/become-a-negotiation-jujitsu-master/

17. ncqa.org/hedis

18. www.cms.gov

19. https://www.healthcare.gov

Chapter 3

Financial Planning

Have you ever prepared a nice concise list for the grocery store only to get home with a ton of things you never intended to buy? What about those times you went for something specific and somehow came home without it? Worse yet, have you ever realized when you got to the store that you didn't bring the list at all? We've all been there. So we all know that planning, adherence, and looking back are critical functions in all areas. It's the same with financial planning – if you only do it at the beginning of the year, pay no attention to it throughout the year, or don't plan at all, you are setting yourself up for failure. Failing to plan is planning to fail.

The first two sections of this book consider cost and revenue. Now let's look at some strategies to prevent theft, manage capital, and more. Throughout this section, make sure you're not only thinking critically but also practically.

3.1 Identifying New Income Sources

The historical notion of revenue generation in healthcare invited the perception of healthcare providers using patients as cattle to fatten their bottom lines. As patients' out-of-pocket expenses continue to rise along with the prioritization of transparency, the public has a greater awareness of what it takes to keep healthcare organizations running.

This awareness creates a newer, savvier patient population with higher expectations. With heightened expectations comes increased responsibility to provide a more favorable healthcare experience.

To fund a 'Next Generation' healthcare experience, we must identify new, alternative, and sustainable income sources. There will be new clinical interventions that may yield a higher rate of return. Most, however, will include additional overhead such as clinical staff, equipment, liability coverage, technology and an educated/certified workforce. Alternative income sources are already available to us, but too many of us don't view these sources as tangible revenue opportunities. Examples of alternative income sources include improved financial oversight, process improvement, and keeping every dollar earned. Income sustainability is a critical component to financial success. As we do our due diligence in keeping our organizations financially viable, we'll want to include strategies that enable long-term success – strategies that withstand the test of time, changing regulations and trends. Sustainable revenue strategies will integrate long-term, proactive approaches with innovations in financial management and care delivery.

Avoiding Revenue Leakage

At its core, revenue leakage is the outcome of unrealized income due to an inability to pinpoint and resolve not only broken touch points but broken processes within an organization. Consider this: your organization had the potential to generate $1.5 million in quarterly revenues, but due to revenue leakage experienced an income shortfall of $100 thousand. Imagine how that income could have been used to fund new equipment, provide pay increases and/or bonuses, procure new technology, pay off loans, build reserves, or strengthen professional services. We could keep going, but the point has been made that revenue leakage impacts patient care, workforce retention and financial standing.

Let's take a look at a handful of common revenue leakage areas and solutions to address them.

Exhibit 3.1 Common Revenue Leakage Touchpoints

Revenue Leakage Touchpoint	Solution
Patient Payments	Patients are more financially savvy regarding online shopping and delivery services. Implement touchless payment options, payment via patient portal, eStatements, pre-visit planning process, patient notification prior to date of service, time of service collections, payment plans for large balances, credit card on file.
Inability to Coordinate Benefits	COB non-payments cannot be passed on by billing the patient. Utilize an insurance discovery tool that queries multiple databases to locate insurance and provide accurate sequencing of primary, secondary and tertiary coverage.
Reconciliation Process	Implement a consistent process that allows for checks, balances and comparisons of notes that are closed, visits that were kept, services rendered against services scheduled.
Payment Fees	This appears to be a typo but you read that right – many of us actually pay to get paid. Opting out of financial arrangements that require a finance fee or other processing fee keeps more money in your organization's pockets. We'll discuss avoiding these tactics below.
Payment Posting Errors	Avoid creating credit balances and duplicate entries that falsely make your Accounts Receivable appear as if monies have been collected but have not. Utilize Electronic Remittance Advice (ERA) and automated payment posting. Include comparison of payments posted to an uploaded fee schedule that will also capture underpayments and overpayments.

The National Association of Healthcare Revenue Integrity defines revenue integrity as the need to "prevent recurrence of issues that can cause revenue leakage and/or compliance risks through effective, efficient, replicable processes and internal controls across the continuum of patient care, supported by the appropriate documentation and the application of sound financial practices that are able to withstand audits at any point in time."[1]

At its core, revenue integrity optimization results in root cause correction and process improvements. A key to revenue integrity is a sound understanding of the revenue cycle processes, including the following:

- Front-end processes, such as patient access and provider credentialing
- Mid-cycle processes, such as documentation, charge capture, and coding
- Back-end processes, including claim production and billing, follow-up and collections, payment review and payer contracts, denial management, and financial and key performance indicator reporting

To minimize revenue leakage through revenue integrity, consider implementing compliance measures, automation of workflows, leadership and staff coaching, ethical business practices in the form of policies and procedures, methods to monitor processes, and data analytics. Stay at the forefront of changes in the healthcare reimbursement and regulatory landscape to refocus or pivot revenue integrity functions based on upcoming changes.

Revenue leakage can be minimized by assessing organizational touchpoints in which revenue is either received or processed. Identify the functions or departments that revenue is received or generated. Educate the individuals who are involved in the revenue cycle to ensure their understanding of core responsibilities that will impact revenue. Create accountability measures that, after revenue leakage is identified, integrate revenue integrity metrics into workflows.

Exhibit 3.2 Revenue Touchpoints

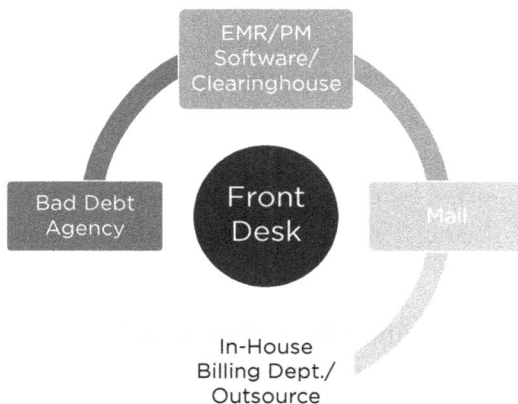

Paying to Get Paid

You might be asking yourself, "Why on Earth would I pay to get paid?" There is a convenience factor that blinds us to how we pay for convenience itself by allowing payers to keep a portion of our payment in exchange for the convenience of using their cards. At the least, the decision to pay for this convenience should be consciously made. The consistent eroding of healthcare reimbursement is only heightened by paying fees to funding sources to accept payment for healthcare services rendered.

These payment terms include a fee to accept the payment. These fees are demonstrated through a finance charge for "Virtual Credit Card Payments" or "VCCs/vPayments". Some insurance companies also have EFT fees.

A virtual credit card (VCC) is a form of payment made by insurance companies to healthcare providers to reimburse for services rendered to beneficiaries. VCCs are not actual credit cards but rather documents that are usually mailed, faxed or electronically sent to the provider. The document contains a credit card number and expiration date along with the payment amount.

Health plans have difficulty keeping up with EFT/ERA enrollments given the large volume of payments that are processed nationally, as well as the large volume of benefit plans within their networks. It's no wonder that health plans find it an administrative benefit to outsource adjudication and claims payment. Now, what if we told you that not only could health plans outsource the administrative burden of claims payment but in addition to that, actually profit from this activity? It's true – health plans may impose a processing or finance charge to the provider and split that monetary value with their Third-Party Administrator (TPA).

Hopefully you're asking yourself, "Well, how are these processing or finance fees being funded?" Glad you asked. Your organization's contractual allowed amount is being decreased. To put it another way: the payment fees are essentially being deducted from your payment. Yes, you have been unwittingly roped into a financial cycle that financially benefits the health plan and their TPA.

Exhibit 3.3 Paying To Get Paid Cycle

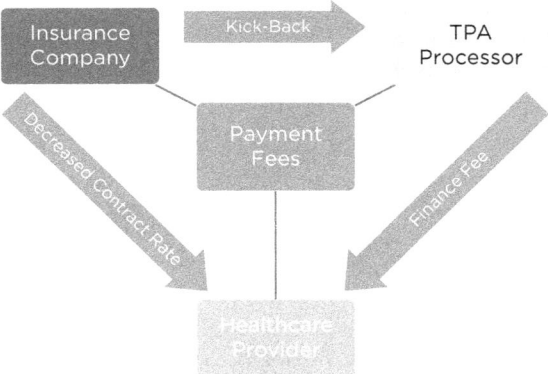

Insurance Company — Kick-Back — TPA Processor

Decreased Contract Rate

Payment Fees

Finance Fee

Healthcare Provider

Seeing that there is no financial upside for healthcare providers to pay to get paid, we can now turn our attention toward solutions. Let's start by asking the question, "When was the last time you audited your payers' profiles and confirmed your organization's pay-to information and pay-to preference?". If it's been a while, stop what you're doing and get started. A good start to initiation of your payer's profile is explained in the following steps:

Audit of Payer Profiles

Review your providers' CAQH, NPI, PECOS and commercial payer portal profile information. Make necessary updates to correspondence addresses, taxonomy codes, authorized official provider and practice demographic information, and most importantly, pay-to address information. Confirm the records for your clearinghouse are up to date. Contact top payers to confirm data from step #1 is correct. If it is not, make those corrections in writing, on practice letterhead. Follow up to ensure updates have been completed on the payer side.

Do not fret, my friend, you have options – yes, you can opt out of these arrangements. You are hereby empowered to say no to paying to get paid. This message is approved by the Centers for Medicare and Medicaid Services (CMS). In Section 1104 of the Affordable

Care Act (ACA), providers may refuse Virtual Credit Card Payments and request either a paper check or an Electronic Funds Transfer (EFT).

Insurance participation agreements, however, may have language that binds organizations into accepting virtual credit card payments or other payment fees. Review your contracts and always opt out of these payment terms. If possible, request carve-outs or negotiate exclusions from payment fees and virtual credit card payments.

Oftentimes, the employee(s) who are receiving payments on behalf of your organization have one goal in mind – to zero out an account balance and stop the aging process. We can all agree that this is a shared goal, but not at the expense of the practice. Unfortunately for an organization's bottom line, tunnel vision and lack of awareness result in agreeing to modified payment terms on behalf of your organization. Having payments posted at the time of receipt, which decreases the ability to monitor incoming payment types, is typical for many medical practices. Whoever is managing the mail/payer incoming correspondence exerts some control over acceptance of VCC payments. Regardless of your practice preference, make sure that you structure your internal controls and processes.

Posting VCCs will highlight the ineffectiveness of paying to get paid. Some practice management software may even recommend against posting VCCs directly in their systems due to inaccuracy of account reconciliation. The typical Explanation of Benefits (EOB) or Electronic Remittance Advice (ERA) will include the allowed amount, contractual adjustments and patient responsibility. VCC EOB/ERA guidance will not be accurate as it includes a finance fee that is deducted from your contracted allowed amount. This amount is not accounted for in your fee schedule or Explanation of Benefits (EOB), a situation that will undoubtedly create a payment posting issue. If your organization is accepting VCCs, how do you track lost revenue as a result of paying VCC finance fees? When reviewing the below EOB, you will see that the VCC finance fee is not included.

Exhibit 3.4 Sample Explanation of Benefits

Sample EOB – Basic

Cutten Mend Health Insurance
Explanation of Benefits

Patient Provider	DOS	Proc	Mod	Billed	Allowed	Pt Resp	Paid	Remark
John Doe Dr. Smith	1/1/2021	99213		100.00	80.00	16.00 10.00	54.00	PR-2, PR-3, CO-45
	1/1/2021	96372	25	25.00	8.00	2.00	6.00	PR-2, CO-45
			TOTAL	125.00	88.00	28.00	60.00	

Remark Codes
PR-2   Patient Coinsurance
PR-3   Patient Copay
CO-45 Charge exceeds maximum allowable

Payment: CHECK
Tracking#: 123456
Date: 1/31/2021

Answer these questions regarding your internal posting process of VCC payments

1. Will you "swipe" through your merchant services device or enter directly into your practice management software?

2. Is your merchant services device interfaced with your PM software?

3. Do you have an adjustment code for the VCC finance fee?

4. Are you keeping a copy of the VCC and attaching it to your daily payment batch or to individual patient accounts?

5. Have you missed the timely payment receipt window to post outdated VCCs?

6. How are you reconciling VCCs to zero out accounts?

By answering the above questions, hopefully it's becoming clearer just how impactful VCC payments are to the financial health and operational efficiency of your organization. This impact is especially evident in fee schedule management as these fees represent a threat to your bottom line.

Let's make a few financial assumptions to demonstrate the negative impact VCC finance fees have on your fee schedule. Looking at Payer #2 below, let's add a 3% VCC finance fee to 30% of payments received over a 6-month timeframe. The financial impact is $10,507.50. With so many financial priorities facing healthcare organizations today, just imagine how those funds could have been spent to improve clinical care, workforce development and debt reduction.

Exhibit 3.5 VCC Finance Fee – Fee Schedule Impact

CPT Codes	Description	Charge	Payer # 1	Payer # 2	Claim Count	VCC Payment Discount
99203	NP L3	145.00	117.01	125.00	1570	$1,766.25
99204	NP L4	220.00	177.92	160.00	1200	$1,728.00
99205	NP L5	250.00	223.39	239.00	1000	$2,151.00
99213	Estab L3	100.00	80.46	70.00	2000	$1,260.00
99214	Estab L4	125.00	117.58	119.00	1750	$1,874.25
99215	Estab L5	150.00	157.40	160.00	1200	$1,728.00
Amount Paid in Virtual Credit Card Fees						**$10,507.50**

Venture Capital

Non-clinical investors are a staple within the healthcare industry. At one point there was concern that the infusion of venture capital (VC) cash into healthcare services would negatively impact care quality, as the initial thinking was that venture capital equals profits over patients. While this concern has not completely disappeared, pay-for-performance is such an integral component of fee-for-service payments that the original widespread concern has diminished. Some states have limitations on non-physician investors within the clinical aspects of the medical organization. Many of these limitations do not include non-medical operations of a medical organization.

To this point, the MSO model is a structure that allows non-physician investors to manage the administrative components of a medical organization, leaving the physicians to have ownership and responsibility over the clinical directorship. There are also liability carrier guidelines that prohibit 51% ownership by non-physicians or non-clinicians. The rationale for liability carriers is risk limitation by ensuring clinical decisions are prioritized within their policy holder's organizations. If your organization is considering cash-flow infusion or venture capitalist acquisition, please take these limitations into consideration.

These non-physician investor/ownership limitations are separate rules from the non-physician practitioner (NPP), advanced practice providers (APP), or mid-level provider ownership guidelines. The same conflict of interest for this group of providers does not exist as it does for the non-physician investors. The states that allow NPPs to own medical practices do so under state-level scope of practice guidelines. This subset of providers who are approved to own medical practices without the requirement of a physician collaborative agreement or direct supervision by a physician will be subject to financial limitations. These financial limitations include but are not limited to insurance participation exclusions and a 15% decrease in fee schedule reimbursement for direct insurance billing. NPPs have the ability to bill "incident-to" a physician and obtain 100% of the physician's insurance allowed amount.

Crunchbase, a company providing business information about private and public companies, including investment and funding information, reports that healthcare venture funding topped $5.7 billion in April 2023. At a time when global venture funding was down 56%, healthcare remained a leader target for VC dollars.[2]

Healthcare organizations considering VC funding or acquisition should position their organizations in a manner that places high priority on regulatory compliance and justifies profitability and scalability while being operationally savvy and demonstrating optimization of technology. VCs leverage consulting firms to perform due diligence on their behalf.

Those who flourish in accessing venture capital funding have been successful in managing and lowering their financial risks. VCs are looking for easy entry, controllable risk, reliance on "clinical experts to do what they know best" and large returns. Healthcare organizations that are run in a manner that demonstrates consistent and future profits are the best candidates for VC partnerships. If your organization is interested in diversifying your financial portfolio, the goal is to position your organization in a manner that is attractive for VC funding.

It's also critical to understand the concrete data VC funding sources use to make their decisions. Consider internally assessing your organization's standings with the following metrics prior to approaching VC for funding. Develop an internal financial pro forma to highlight your organization's financial strengths and opportunities that would be attractive to a VC.

Financial metrics to internally assess prior to or in preparation for venture capital funding:

1. Net Collections Ratio
2. Aging Accounts Receivable
3. Productivity – CPT/HCPCS, Provider, Site
4. Payer Mix
5. Gross Charges, Adjustments and Net Collections
6. Profit & Loss
7. Balance Sheet
8. Payer Mix
9. MIPS, AAPM, HEDIS and/or scoring
10. Grouped Denials

Moving in the VC direction should not be seen as a short-term business strategy. Venture capital funding is a long-term financial model that should be strategically incorporated into your current business plan. Many of our business plans have shifted as a result of COVID-19, the Public Health Emergency (PHE) and the Great Resignation. As you prepare to engage in VC funding, circle back to your original business plan to identify shifts in your organization. Use your business plan components as a checklist to analyze clinical care, finances, operations, technology and compliance factors that may impact your standing with a VC.

Exhibit 3.6 Business Plan Analysis

BP Focus Area	Current Status	Strategic Goal	Activities Required	KPI/Benchmarks
Mission Statement				
Description of Business				
Company Ownership/ Legal Entity				
Location				
Hours of Operation				
Products and Services				
Suppliers				
Leadership/Governance				
Financial Management				
Start-Up/Acquisition Summary				

Leveraging VC funding might be a good strategy for your organization. Conduct your due diligence to see if it's a good fit for you. It's also OK to be very selective of your VC partner to ensure long-term strategic and organizational cultural alignment. More and more VCs are identifying the value of entry into healthcare. Many interested VCs place a high priority on technology, which makes medical organizations who are maximizing technology for care delivery, billing, financial oversight, security and operational efficiency very appealing. Consider utilizing the below Healthcare Financial Management Association (HFMA) tool for a smooth VC process.[3]

Checklist for an effective venture capital process:

- Do we have diverse ventures from multiple channels?
- Are line managers involved in the selection process?
- Is there a clearly defined vetting process for deals?
- Do we have a process for identifying and grooming venture champions?

- Are there frequent forecast updates to support tactical shifts?
- Is there a process for addressing pilot pain points?
- Is there a roll-out plan for implementation that balances need and speed of execution?
- Are we developing a culture of continuous improvement?

Venture and external capital may be a positive funding factor for healthcare organizations. To avoid negotiating from a position of weakness, fix any internal financial or operational messes prior to engaging external funding. It's always a good idea to regularly perform a practice and financial assessment to gauge organizational financial health. When developing a financial pro forma, pull in your business plan and highlight key team members who bring operational value to your organization.

Preparing for a Successful Due Diligence Process

Interest continues to increase from external funding via venture capital investors and private equity firms. This rise could be attributed to technology advancements, care delivery innovations and population health models that open opportunities for investors to realize financial gains in healthcare. As this interest continues to rise, healthcare organizations are best served by understanding and mastering the due diligence process to protect their interests in these transactions.

Healthcare due diligence traditionally assesses financial performance and legal liabilities. During financial due diligence, independent financial firms review and evaluate balance sheets, income statements, audit reports, cash flow statements, and other financial documents, as well as potential changes in legislation, regulation and market forces; generally, to measure and project financial performance. Prior to information sharing, both parties will ensure documentation is in place to outline levels of access and information required to complete the transaction. Healthcare organizations typically prepare for external entities accessing their data by identifying the information to be shared and reviewed. In legal due diligence, attorneys examine the following factors of the presenting entity:

1. Structures
2. Business permits and/or approvals
3. Employment and labor law matters
4. Environmental law approvals and permits
5. Contractual rights and obligations
6. Intellectual property rights and obligations

Additionally, attorneys may focus on real estate matters, securities, and financing regulatory compliance, tax exposure risks, consumer protection laws and exposure risks, and previous and/or current litigation. Healthcare organizations that keep good records and address action items related to each of the above factors of their facilities, operations and governance will be prepared for a smooth due diligence process.

Governance, risk, and compliance-related due diligence is sensitive and complicated across healthcare, because providers, payers, and their suppliers are subject to a tremendous number of federal and state laws and regulations that govern their services and products. The additional complication comes in when multiple laws and regulations overlap, supersede or contradict one another.

As a result of these complexities, purchasers can inherit significant regulatory liabilities and costs, including the loss of future revenues without a complete and in-depth understanding of potential purchases. This is particularly sensitive where purchasers are considering investments into existing entities, or stock purchases where liabilities follow ownership interests. Healthcare organizations that itemize, solve for, and effectively mitigate these risks are in a superior position for consideration of external funding.

By performing proper due diligence, purchasers can:

1. Identify and assess regulatory and legal risks related to the target company
2. Evaluate the regulatory strengths and weaknesses of target company, and measure the past, current and future

operational and financial effects of those strengths and weaknesses

3. Confirm and, where necessary, redetermine a realistic value/price for the target company

4. Identify issues that must be addressed prior to closing, including in transactions documents, where appropriate

This due diligence work provides invaluable insights that inform go/no-go decisions, establishes a post-transaction work plan, and ensures sufficient escrow. It also allows healthcare organizations to leverage results to institute corrective actions for sustainability and future financial opportunities.

Governance, risk, and compliance due diligence should identify material gaps in compliance with applicable healthcare laws and regulations, measure the financial and operational effects of the goals, identify effective corrective and preventive action plans, project the costs of these plans, and mitigate buyers' liability exposures.

While the appropriateness and depth of governance, risk, and compliance due diligence will vary depending on the transaction, the following areas could be subject to reasonable governance, risk, and compliance due diligence in the acquisition of any healthcare company. With this scrutiny in mind, healthcare organizations that are considering external investments are well-served in developing an internal due diligence roadmap to prepare for such a process.

Healthcare Organization Internal Due Diligence Roadmap

1. The management of the healthcare revenue cycle from beginning to end, with a particular focus on healthcare services and delivery, claims development and submission matters, including the medical necessity of services, documentation, coding and billing under Federal and payer standards, including the federal **False Claims Act**.[4]

2. The management of financial relationships with sources of business or referrals, including matters under the federal **Anti-Kickback Statute**.[5]

3. The management of self-referral arrangements, including matters under the **Federal Physician Self-Referral Law**, widely known as Stark Law.[6]

4. The management of financial relationships with patients, including matters under the **Federal Civil Monetary Penalties Law**.[7]

5. Employee and contractor vetting against the **US Department of Health and Human Services, Office of the Inspector General**'s List of Excluded Individuals/Entities, the **Government Services Administration**'s List of Debarred or Suspended Persons, and the **U.S. Department of the Treasury's Office of Foreign Asset Control**'s List of Specially Designated National or Blocked Persons.[8]

6. The management of applicable licensing, credentialing, registration, permit and accreditation requirements under each specific authority

7. The management of environmental, health and safety requirements under applicable **Federal Occupational, Safety and Health Administration** requirements (Occupational Safety and Health Standards, 1910).[9]

8. The management of the confidentiality and availability of patient information, including matters under the **Federal Health Insurance Portability and Accountability Act of 1996** (as amended from time to time, "HIPAA"), including all pertinent regulations set forth in Title 45, Parts 160 and 164 of the Code of Federal Regulations issued by the **U.S. Department of Health and Human Services, Office of Civil Rights** as either have been amended by Subtitle D of the Health Information Technology for Economic and Clinical Health Act of 2009 ("HITECH Act"). This assessment should include an assessment of the target organizations' compliance with HIPAA's administrative, physical and technical requirements, including a cyber-security assessment against

the standards of the **National Institute of Standards in Technology** (NIST) or a similar HIPAA-compliant professional standard

9. The structure and effectiveness of the target organizations' confidential information privacy and security programs under the standards of the **US Department of Justice** and the **US Department of Health and Human Services, Office of Civil Rights,** including leadership and communication, risk assessments, policies and procedures, training, measuring and monitoring or activities, internal investigations, corrective and preventive actions, along with any litigation, administrative or regulatory proceedings, investigations, or government actions, and related insurance coverages. Where applicable, management of the requirements of relevant state-specific corporate practice of medicine requirements

10. The structure and effectiveness of the target organizations' healthcare corporate governance and compliance programs under the standards of the **US Department of Justice** and the **US Department of Health and Human Services, Office of Inspector General,** including leadership and communication, risk assessments, policies and procedures, training, measuring and monitoring or activities, internal investigations, corrective and preventive actions, along with any related litigation, administrative or regulatory proceedings, investigations, or government actions, and related insurance coverages

11. The structure and effectiveness of the target organizations' legal risk management programs, including leadership and communication, risk assessments, policies and procedures, training, measuring and monitoring or activities, internal investigations, corrective and preventive actions, along with any litigation, administrative or regulatory proceedings, investigations, or government actions, and related insurance coverages.

When conducted at an early stage, this work better allows investors and healthcare entities involved in these transactions to make well-informed decisions, including appropriate adjustments to transaction terms.

The authors would like to thank Jeffrey Miller, J.D., Director-in-Charge, Granite GRC, for collaborating with us on this topic.

Federal and State Funding / Certifications

Most funding received by healthcare providers and related facilities is derived from insurance reimbursement and successful value-based program participation. It's financially sound to diversify healthcare funding sources outside of the typical previously described actors. Diversifying funding sources involves understanding your organization's core competencies, board specialties, resources, skill set, technology and capacity to apply for Federal, State and local funding opportunities.

The Small Business Administration (SBA) was a key resource for healthcare organizations for PPE assistance during the COVID-19 Public Health Emergency (PHE). The SBA has funding opportunities that healthcare organizations should consider leveraging. There are also federal population health grants that should be considered. The Centers for Disease Control and Prevention (CDC) for many years has funded the Improving the Health of Americans through Prevention and Management of Diabetes, Heart Disease and Stroke grant (CDC-RFA-DP18-1815). This ongoing grant is awarded to State Health Departments to prevent or delay the development of type 2 diabetes and cardiovascular disease in people at high risk, and to improve the health of people living with diabetes.[10]

Although these federal funds are awarded to state health departments, private practices and healthcare facilities may collaborate on these initiatives to align with state entities and play a role in population health and chronic disease management. These agencies benefit from the insight offered by private practices and health systems, especially if adapted to agile and flexible care delivery.

Exhibit 3.7 CDC Funding[11]

State	Diabetes	Heart Disease and Stroke	Total Award
Alabama	$932,302	$932,302	$1,864,604
Alaska	$732,655	$732,655	$1,465,310
Arizona	$945,509	$945,509	$1,891,018
Arkansas	$906,189	$906,189	$1,812,378
California	$1,356,623	$1,356,623	$2,713,246
Colorado	$820,919	$820,919	$1,641,838
Connecticut	$772,132	$772,132	$1,544,264
Delaware	$772,607	$772,607	$1,545,214
District of Columbia	$899,392	$899,392	$1,798,784
Florida	$1,104,864	$1,104,864	$2,209,728
Georgia	$986,725	$986,725	$1,973,450
Hawaii	$734,425	$734,425	$1,468,850
Idaho	$821,761	$821,761	$1,643,522
Illinois	$961,011	$961,011	$1,922,022
Indiana	$894,592	$894,592	$1,789,184
Iowa	$801,055	$801,055	$1,602,110
Kansas	$807,631	$807,631	$1,615,262
Kentucky	$945,851	$945,851	$1,891,702
Louisiana	$986,282	$986,282	$1,972,564
Maine	$787,634	$787,634	$1,575,268
Maryland	$802,215	$802,215	$1,604,430
Massachusetts	$828,880	$828,880	$1,657,760
Michigan	$958,021	$958,021	$1,916,042
Minnesota	$799,198	$799,198	$1,598,396
Mississippi	$980,243	$980,243	$1,960,486
Missouri	$887,071	$887,071	$1,774,142
Montana	$805,045	$805,045	$1,610,090
Nebraska	$776,164	$776,164	$1,552,328
Nevada	$845,111	$845,111	$1,690,222
New Hampshire	$696,095	$696,095	$1,392,190
New Jersey	$856,632	$856,632	$1,713,264

State	Diabetes	Heart Disease and Stroke	Total Award
New Mexico	$930,578	$930,578	$1,861,156
New York	$1,092,787	$1,092,787	$2,185,574
North Carolina	$970,807	$970,807	$1,941,614
North Dakota	$744,572	$744,572	$1,489,144
Ohio	$973,707	$973,707	$1,947,414
Oklahoma	$897,780	$897,780	$1,795,560
Oregon	$847,533	$847,533	$1,695,066
Pennsylvania	$958,821	$958,821	$1,917,642
Rhode Island	$803,290	$803,290	$1,606,580
South Carolina	$896,640	$896,640	$1,793,280
South Dakota	$792,836	$792,836	$1,585,672
Tennessee	$929,920	$929,920	$1,859,840
Texas	$1,221,421	$1,221,421	$2,442,842
Utah	$770,663	$770,663	$1,541,326
Vermont	$758,303	$758,303	$1,516,606
Virginia	$860,905	$860,905	$1,721,810
Washington	$851,100	$851,100	$1,702,200
West Virginia	$903,714	$903,714	$1,807,428
Wisconsin	$839,825	$839,825	$1,679,650
Wyoming	$749,965	$749,965	$1,499,930
Total Award	**$45,000,001**	**$45,000,001**	**$90,000,002**

State business certification sets your organization down the path of exclusivity for accessing state-based procurement opportunities only available to certified businesses located in the state. The purpose of state-based certification is to elevate organizations who have met state criteria, which includes being located in the state, having met financial thresholds and successful completion of unique application processes. Some healthcare organizations may be deemed above the financial threshold for eligibility, but each state and certification requirement will vary. There are three state-based certifications we will review, and healthcare organizations that meet the certifications' criteria may wish to consider. Check with your state to see if similar certification opportunities exist.

Exhibit 3.8 State-based Certifications

State	Certification	Online Procurement Portal and Sample Procurement Opportunity	State-Based Certification Office
Maryland	Minority Business Enterprise (MBE), Disadvantaged Business Enterprise (DBE), Small Business Enterprise (SBE), Airport Concessions Disadvantaged Business Enterprise (ACDBE)	[12] -Ryan White Medical Services	Maryland Department of Transportation (MDOT)
Massachusetts	Minority Business Enterprise (MBE), Women Business Enterprise (WBE), Veteran Business Enterprise (VBE), Portuguese Business Enterprise (PBE)	COMMBUYS [13] -Influenza Vaccine	Supplier Diversity Office (SDO)
Washington, DC	Certified Business Enterprise (CBE)	[14] -Medical Services, Physical Examinations	DC Department of Small and Local Business Development (DSLBD)

3.2 Investing in Your Practice

With the turbulence of the financial markets, investments can seem scary, but there are ways to invest in your organization with both short- and long-term opportunities for success. In healthcare, these can be anything from new imaging machines to construction of entire healthcare facilities. The key for investments is to evaluate the potential for success, performance opportunities (likely worst-case and optimal), and the time it will take to break even (two, three, or five years). To be clear, in this section we aren't talking about stocks and bonds; that's a whole different book! Let's kick things off with investments that can be quickly implemented.

Some short-term investments include opportunities like technology upgrades that can provide a quick boost to revenue, improve practice operations, enhance efficiency, or increase patient satisfaction. These investments are typically more necessity-based and include the following:

- Older technology no longer meeting interoperability requirements
- Newer software offering greater data analysis
- Software that supports the provision of new services (like telehealth)
- Televisions for waiting rooms that improve the patient experience
- Upgrading phone systems and call centers to improve operational efficiency as well as patient satisfaction

These types of practice investments can be predictable and will not carry on from year to year though they may recur in longer cycles like every three or five years. Preparing for these events can help practices to quickly execute when needs arise.

Need-based investments assist healthcare organizations with meeting internal and external demands for operational improvements as well as enhanced workforce and patient experiences. Investments and upgrades to internal infrastructure such as technology, telephone systems and software may seem like expensive investments; however, when you factor in the operational improvements as a result of these investments, the return on investment is there.

For the private practice arena, the most common type of longer-term investment seen is practice ownership, whether that is starting a new practice, investing in an existing practice, or working your way toward a portion of physician ownership in the practice. When considering practice ownership, consider state ownership requirements prior to entering into ownership agreements. States that have licensure requirements will need to be consulted to determine which provider types have approval for clinical practice ownership. States with full practice authority have approved legislation for nurse practitioners to own medical practices without a physician collaborative agreement. There are also states that prohibit non-physician, non-clinical individuals from having majority ownership of medical practices. This law seeks to exclude investors and other non-clinicians from having authority over the clinical operations of a healthcare facility.

There are other opportunities as well, such as investing in ambulatory surgery centers, dialysis centers, or other ancillary revenue sources that can provide long-term residual income. The investment opportunities also need to take Anti-Trust, Stark Law and Anti-Kickback with the related Safe-Harbors into consideration. Investors want to avoid the appearance of "pay-to-play" so be sure that corporate structures are such that these appearances are not factors.

Whenever you are considering a long-term investment of this nature, it is highly recommended to consult a CPA, your legal counsel, and any other professionals who can guide you in best practice processes and realistic expectations. Keep in mind that ownership does not simply equate to revenue. Having ownership in a practice may mean that during a challenging financial time, you are called upon to help support payroll or cosign on loans. There is accountability and responsibility with ownership interests, so they are not something to be considered lightly.

Health System Investments in Private Practice

Integrated care delivery and value-based payment models have upended the original Physician Self-Referral law, which was geared toward combating overutilization in a fee-for-service payment structure. Now that CMS payments are tied to outcomes, care collaboration is vital for economic success. Permitting legal care collaboration required some retooling of the original Physician Self-Referral/ Stark Law. This reengineering allows hospital systems, physician practices and other qualified stakeholders to financially collaborate without running afoul of Stark Law by having financial relationships that are qualified as value-based activities, value-based arrangements, and value-based enterprises. The following qualifying start-up financial arrangements between these stakeholders include:[15]

- Infrastructure creation and provision
- Network development and management, including the configuration of a correct ambulatory network and the restructuring of existing providers and suppliers to provide efficient care
- Care coordination mechanisms, including care coordination processes across multiple organizations
- Clinical management systems
- Quality improvement mechanisms including a mechanism to improve patient experience of care
- Creation of governance and management structure
- Care utilization management, including chronic disease management, limiting hospital readmissions, creation of care protocols, and patient education
- Creation of incentives for performance-based payment systems and the transition from fee-for-service payment system to one of shared risk of losses
- Hiring of new staff, including care coordinators (including nurses, technicians, physicians, and/or non-physician practitioners), umbrella organization management, quality leadership, analytical team, liaison team, IT support, financial management, contracting, and risk management
- IT, including EHR systems, electronic health information exchanges that allow for electronic data exchange across multiple platforms, data reporting systems (including all payer claims data reporting systems), and data analytics (including staff and systems, such as software tools, to perform such analytic functions)
- Consultant and other professional support, including market analysis for antitrust review, legal services, and financial and accounting services
- Organization and staff training costs
- Incentives to attract primary care physicians
- Capital investments, including loans, capital contributions, grants, and withholds. Many of these activities similarly facilitate a value-based enterprise's (and its VBE participants')

transition from health care delivery and payment mechanisms based on the volume of items and services provided to mechanisms based on the quality of care and control of care costs for a target patient population.

Many healthcare organizations could benefit from a financial infusion within the above areas of their organizations. Confirming qualifications, needs and interest with health systems will set you on a positive path to avoiding Stark Law issues while collaboratively managing patient populations. Many health systems are motivated to provide the above financial investments to reduce unnecessary readmissions by financially supporting community physician practices without breaking laws.

Although we have this new financial latitude, the concept of fair market value hasn't gone away. HHS "modified the definition drawn from §413.134(b)(2) to include analogous provisions for determining the fair market value of any items or services, including personal services, employment relationships, and rental arrangements."[16]

Adequately Prepare for Operational Changes Based on New Technology Investments

Consider the following: Allison B. is the practice administrator for a mid-sized primary care practice in Arlington, VA, which sees approximately 80-90 patients per day. There was a challenge in the facility which required transitioning to Voice over IP (VoIP) services for its phone systems. This created another challenge as leaders did not fully understand the objective of the transition to VoIP or the features associated with the new platform.

To solve for this, the organization dedicated time to educate team members and to ask critical questions of the new vendor. This allowed the practice to more effectively use its phone system and teach staff about beneficial features of the new technology.

As a result of this investment and implementation strategy, the facility realized:

- A decrease in patient complaints
- A decrease in repeated phone calls
- A direct line for every staff member
- The ability to access the phone lines remotely (advanced call features)
- Voicemails that can be transcribed to email
- The ability to have an automated attendant answers phone calls and route them to the right person or department

On average, the monthly cost to the organization is $1,250 for 28 lines and well worth the money.

Leadership: Allison B., Practice Administrator
Location: Arlington, VA
# of Providers: 8
Specialty: Primary Care

3.3 Managing Working Capital

Surely you've heard the phrase, 'Cash is king," but let's challenge that with a quote from Derek Shaw, President of Invicta Health Solutions, who coined the phrase, "Cash is queen." This quote is derived from the concept that the queen is the most powerful and versatile object on a chessboard. The ability of the queen to defend and attack is similar to the ability of having cash on hand to defend organizations from unexpected financial needs and attack by leveraging that cash for growth and expansion. Effectively managing working capital starts with the availability of cash.

The formula for working capital is:

Current Assets – Current Liabilities = Working Capital

Assessing current versus long-term assets in the working capital formula is critical, as current assets are an indication of short-term availability of assets, whereas long-term assets have a historical value that is not typically used to fund day-to-day operations. Long-term assets such as real-estate, facilities/property, medical equipment, and even patient lists have value but are not typically immediately available for cash conversion. Short-term assets are typically recovered within twelve months and are generally cash-convertible within a year. Remember, cash is queen, so we want the largest portion of current assets convertible to cash ASAP!

Over-the-counter Cash Management

Varying industries have specific liquid (easily convertible to cash) assets such as sales, inventory, accounts receivable, money market funds, and cash on hand. Unless your healthcare organization is selling durable medical equipment (DME), inventory may not be a significant liquid asset on your chessboard. Over-the-counter cash received in retail is a fairly straightforward transaction – the cost for goods or services is published and paid by the customer. That same transaction in healthcare organizations is more complex. Publishing healthcare costs and transparency is mandated; for some, however, it's still lacking. Also, the cash payment might be a shared expense requiring verification and calculation of patient responsibility for fees such as copayments, coinsurance, deductibles, self-pay, and other out-of-pocket expenses. Copayment amounts will vary based on the type of specialty services being rendered. As copayment amounts are determined by a patient's insurance benefits, these variances on out-of-pocket expenses will have an impact on an organization's cash on hand. These out-of-pocket amounts vary based on specialty and will run between $20 – $60. One solution to capturing this revenue is to confirm insurance benefits and coverage to determine the true amount owed by patients. This should be done prior to services being rendered and communicated to patients in advance to enable time of service (TOS) payment. It's also important to factor in related costs for collecting this revenue. Mailing patient statements and other labor-intensive functions cut into profit margins, which should drive healthcare organizations to automation of these processes.

With the exception of concierge-type models in which patients expect to pay cash for care, the remaining patient base are insured and have an expectation that their premium-paid coverage will take care of their medical expenses. Over-the-counter cash management requires improving patients' awareness of their financial responsibilities as well as leveraging accurate out-of-pocket expense data. Designing a proactive approach to cash management allows organizations to limit the need to rely on patients for financial information. One strategy for managing over-the-counter cash receipts is to leverage insurance discovery for patients who may have insurance coverage but are either unaware or poorly communicate coverage with your staff. Insurance discovery technology searches for primary, secondary, and tertiary coverage for self-pay in multiple commercial and government payer databases.

With an insurance identification hit rate that averages 39%, insurance discovery products are relevant with healthcare providers because this technology easily verifies vital demographic information in real time. A few of the demographic elements that require validation for clean claims include: name, address, phone number, and social security number.

Advanced algorithms in this type of technology do the heavy lifting, searching multiple databases to find active billable coverage all through one inquiry. As we prioritize workflow enhancement, removing manual validation processes and replacing them with this type of technology increases cash collections. Senior vice president of product management at Inovalon, Karly Rowe, said, "Technology helps providers manage over-the-counter cash and ensure more reimbursements by discovering all applicable coverage, including managed care and advantage replacement plans. It also shows lists of relevant plan types like HMO or PPO."

Accounts Receivable Management

If you've ever heard the authors spill their guts about the importance of Accounts Receivable (A/R) management, feel free to skim through this section. It's no secret that A/R is one of if not the most significant assets to a healthcare organization. The longer A/R ages, the longer your organization waits to tap into that asset. Let's take a look at our Working Capital formula again, factoring our Accounts Receivable as the primary current asset:

**Current Assets – Current Liabilities =
Net Working Capital**

Effective and timely management of accounts receivable will impact net working capital. There are expenses related to managing A/R that should be taken into consideration for overall working capital management. Questions to ask and answer are:

1. Are we leveraging technology to replace or minimize human touchpoints that could be automated with a greater return?

2. What fees are associated with claims processing that could either be eliminated, produced in bulk or negotiated down?

3. Do we provide effective training and supportive resources for staff responsible for A/R coordination to ensure we are following all payer's reimbursement guidelines?

4. How effective is each account touch? Are staff touching accounts multiple times with little to no resolution?

5. Is our payer mix primarily made up of payers with complex or confusing payment guidelines?

Strategies to manage A/R for working capital include reduction of account touches to resolution. The organization cuts into claim profitability each time an account is touched but not resolved. Denials, rejections and non-payments should not only be resolved, but a response plan should be put in place to ensure the same denial does not reoccur. Each time the same denial reoccurs, we create future cash-flow disruption by allowing the same non-payment factor to continue plaguing our A/R as an asset.

Profit and Loss Statement

There are a number of methods to track and trend working capital. The profit and loss (P&L) statement is an effective way to monitor assets and liabilities. Oftentimes this statement is reviewed monthly, quarterly and annually along with the balance sheet. The P&L indicates cash received (assets), expenses (liabilities) and working capital (net revenue). Managing accounts payable can improve working capital by ensuring bill payments are timely and additional fees are reduced. If your EMR does not have an inventory control solution, consider identifying a platform that will track and manage supplies for re-purchasing, create bulk discounts, and avoid expedited shipping fees due to low or no-stock inventory. It's best to be prepared rather than pay extra fees for medical supplies, pharmaceuticals and other care delivery necessities.

Every business has the same goal – make sure you have enough working capital to cover expenses. As you monitor and analyze your working capital, identify the points that create bottlenecks so they may be resolved and monitored over time. There are times within every company's lifecycle when liabilities are greater than assets, but that should not be the norm. Root out cash-flow obstacles and remain diligent by precluding their reoccurence.

3.4 Preventive Management of Rising Charity Spending

In healthcare, charity expenses come with the territory. It's a fact that at some point we will all have charitable write-offs. But even expected situations benefit from optimization and preventive management. So how do we preventively manage expenses that we seemingly have no control over? Like every area where we want to achieve prevention, our first step is to identify the root cause of our charitable expenditures.

Facilities spend anywhere from 0.69% to 2.73% of their budget on charity care.[17] While this might not seem significant at first glance, when coupled with the fact that margins for healthcare facilities are already low, it becomes much more important. Becker's Health reported in 2021 that "Not including federal relief aid, hospital operating margins remained narrow in March at just 1.4 percent."[18] This means that it is quite feasible for a facility to spend more on charity care than they expect to receive as net profit.

How Does Charity Care Differ from Bad Debt?

The terms "charity care" and "bad debt" start off on the same road but get off at different exits. In both cases, they refer to a facility not receiving payment for services rendered. In cases of charity care, this is due to the inability of the patient to pay, most likely because of financial hardship. In contrast, bad debt generally refers to cases where patients *have* the ability to pay but lack the desire to do so. There are times when patients end up in the bad-debt column when they truly don't have the ability to pay for services and should be considered charity care. The method to differentiate between the two is also a wonderful method for establishing a charity care management plan.

The Steps to Charity Care Management

To manage charity care you need to create processes which support the identification of patients with financial hardship, the prevention of increased expenses for these patients, and the coordination with other facilities and social support services to ensure that referral or refusal of services will not result in patient harm.

Identification

With the opacity of the healthcare billing cycle, it's no surprise that legislation like the No Surprises Act was passed. Most patients do not understand their financial obligations for healthcare or what the expenses of certain services could amount to. It is incumbent upon healthcare providers and supporting staff to help inform patients. The benefit is increased insight into the patient's ability to pay. To improve price transparency in your organization, consider employing the following strategies:

- Include a section on your financial policy and new patient paperwork that informs patients of the price ranges for certain services with/without insurance.
- Offer price transparency calculators on your practice website.
- During the visit check-in process, include an opportunity for patients to document their financial concerns and connect them to your billing department
- Make it easy, confidential, and non-judgmental for patients to discuss financial concerns privately.
- Prepare patient educational documents using friendly literate terms.
- Use patient portals as a method to reach out to discuss patient financials.

Prevention

- Provide estimates to patients <u>before</u> services are rendered
  - This is a requirement under the No Surprises Act if you are providing out-of-network services to self-pay patients, patients without insurance, or patients who decline to use their insurance
  - Estimates to patients should give a clear expectation of what is expected of them financially
- Employ trained financial counselors
  - These individuals should be trained in eligibility and benefits verifications
  - They should understand how to evaluate balances of deductibles as well as responsibilities related to coinsurance or copayments
  - They should be scheduled to meet with all patients prior to scheduling of large-cost services such as surgeries and in-office testing/procedures.
- Create a protocol around estimates and education
  - The provision of education and touchpoints for estimates and financial discussions should be built into the timeline for the patient's care cycle
  - New patients should meet with the financial counselor regarding potential costs of future services
  - Payment plans should be standardized and known by all who speak to the patient about billing
  - Financial hardship forms and the criteria for approval should be standardized, mathematical and require documentation

Service Coordination

Patient outcomes and treatment adherence are directly impacted by patients' social determinants of health. Discuss patients' social situations to inform if they are at risk for falling into bad debt or charity care.

- Transportation – Patients with transportation challenges who may not come to preventive appointments as often as they should, or miss scheduled appointments
- Education – Patients with a lower level of formal education or those who may not understand industry-specific terms, financial healthcare processes, or even their treatment plan
- Financial – Patients with low income, high expenses, or other financial hardship
- Nutrition – Patients with challenges accessing food and nutrition
- Language – Patients who have difficulty speaking the language primarily spoken at the facility and by its providers and staff
- Housing – Patients who have housing challenges or uncertainty

Work with your community services to identify opportunities for support. Industry examples of supporting services can be a referral to outside services, collaboration with another facility, and other unique solutions that fit your facility.

Exhibit 3.9 SDOH Barriers and Solutions

SDOH Barrier	Possible Solutions
Transportation	Coordinating with Uber, Lyft or other transportation services to provide low-cost rides for patients to improve appointment attendance.
Education	Create health-literate documents which clearly explain the billing process, the care process, and consider posting videos which explain self-care methods.
Financial	Employ financial counselors and work with patients to identify their income, expenses, and options for care. Collaborate with non-profits, community care centers, and other low-cost opportunities for patients.
Nutrition	Keep a list of local community support centers like food banks, state aid, and community cafeterias.
Language	Consider bilingual staff, deploy the use of remote interpreters via telehealth, use new technology to live translate communications in varied dialects.
Housing	Maintain a list of housing support opportunities including shelters, halfway houses, and other forms of temporary lodging. Become familiar with the processes or the correct contacts for the patient to reach out to.

When patients have barriers to care such as the ones listed above, patients can incur unnecessary cost due to a variety of reasons:

- Inability to understand the costs they are incurring
- Waiting to seek care until their conditions have exacerbated
- Failing to meet treatment plan requirements
- Inability to get to appointments required to keep chronic conditions stable

Putting protocols in place ahead of time will help to avoid rising costs and to ensure that the patients receiving charitable care write-offs are truly the patients in need of that benefit.

Obtaining Cost of Charity Care

AHA provides calculations to identify the cost of charitable care and bad debt:[19]

- Uncompensated Care Charges = Bad Debt Charges + Charity Care Charges
- Cost-to-charge Ratio = Total Expenses Exclusive of Bad Debt / (Gross Patient Revenue + Other Operating Revenue)
- Uncompensated Care Costs = Uncompensated Care Charges x Cost-to-charge Ratio

These calculations are important to note and to evaluate regularly against industry benchmarks for like-sized facilities in similar geographic regions. Evaluate your charity care program annually and build a culture of continuous improvement with existing staff so they can help identify opportunities to improve the program over time.

3.5 Financial Service Line Management

Overseeing financial management at healthcare organizations includes integrating financial success with managing service lines. These service lines have varying risks and expenses, changing regulations, shifting technology, and patient expectations. MHA Online describes a service line as "a way of defining a specific line of business, often inclusive of operational, financial, and strategic attributes, and organizing that line of business with a governance structure. In other industries outside of healthcare, this is known as a product line."[20]

As we integrate the concept of service line management into the financial oversight of healthcare organizations, let's imagine that all U.S.-based healthcare organizations represent one large multi-specialty practice. Within this practice, we have every medical subspecialty.

Each of these service lines has a unique approach to care delivery, patient care needs, equipment, space utilization, technology, billing complexity, workforce certification/skill set, and cost – there are many other factors but, again, this is a fake national multi-specialty practice, so work with us here. Now let's apply this "fake national service line model" to an individual organization. Healthcare organizations need to determine their number of service lines as well as best practices for managing each.

Exhibit 3.10 Multi-Specialty Medical Practice

Service Line	Volume	Acuity Level
Primary Care Services	High	Low
Cardiology Services	Medium	High
Sleep Medicine Services	Low	Medium

Now that we've defined our service lines, let's dig into the details of these encounters and episodes of care. Organizations with multiple service lines may also see the need for multi-disciplinary care for unique patients traveling within the organization. A patient who presents for a routine physical exam by their primary care provider (PCP) may receive a routine EKG. In the event that the EKG is abnormal, that patient might be referred to the cardiologist for further work-up, only to discover that the patient might suffer from sleep apnea requiring a sleep study.

Organizations are tasked with the responsibility of trying to manage all patient care needs under one roof or referring patients out as needed. In our example, it will take internal coordination to ensure that this patient matriculates throughout the organization in a timely manner, with necessary appointments scheduled, handoffs/ referrals to the next provider, bi-directional communication between all providers involved using an interoperable technology platform that allows for medical record documentation to be available to all parties.

There's a saying that it costs money to make money. Providing healthcare is no exception. Two of the prominent service line costs are direct and indirect costs. Direct costs are easier to manage as they tie directly to services such as provider salaries and healthcare supplies. A successful financial model will avoid the exclusion or estimation of indirect costs and rather seek to identify and account for indirect costs within the financial model. According to the National Institutes of Health (NIH) Office of Acquisition Management and Policy (OAMP), indirect costs are "[t]hose costs not readily identified with a specific project or organizational activity but incurred for the joint benefit of both projects and other activities." Indirect service line or "overhead" costs include but are not limited to:[21]

- Rent, lease
- Utilities
- Administrative staff salaries
- Health insurance, retirement plans, FICA taxes, paid leave, holiday pay
- Legal and accounting
- Depreciation

Financial service line management should be done by the individual responsible for overseeing, approving and making decisions about service line expenses. Outsourcing this responsibility to others outside of the cost or service center adds barriers for those not involved in hands-on oversight of potential cost variations such as direct or indirect costs occurring at the service center level. Service center leaders have the capability to manage cost variations; this is at the center of service line financial management.

Exhibit 3.11 Full Consumption Costing and Clinical Variation[22]

Full Consumption Costing and Clinical Variation
Lumbar Spinal Fusion (n=852)

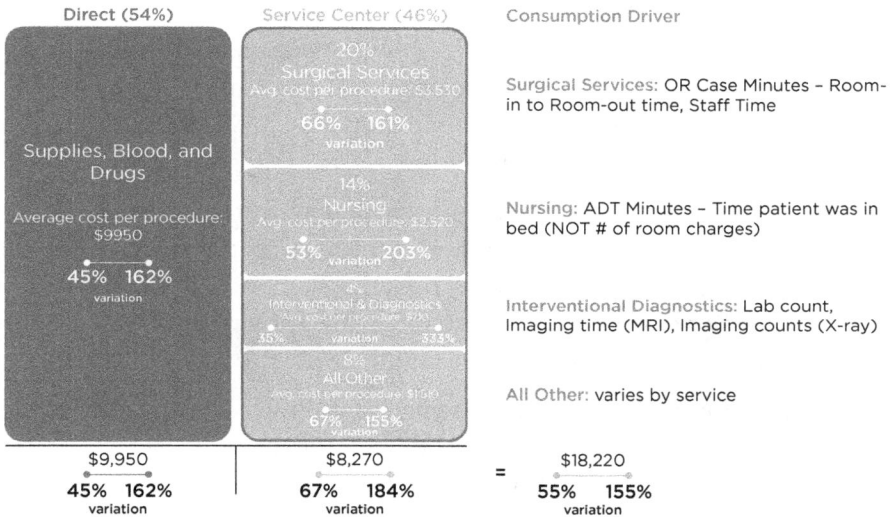

Direct (54%)	Service Center (46%)	Consumption Driver
	20% Surgical Services Avg. cost per procedure: $3,530 66% 161% variation	Surgical Services: OR Case Minutes – Room-in to Room-out time, Staff Time
Supplies, Blood, and Drugs Average cost per procedure: $9950 45% 162% variation	14% Nursing Avg. cost per procedure: $2,520 53% variation 203%	Nursing: ADT Minutes – Time patient was in bed (NOT # of room charges)
	4% Interventional & Diagnostics Avg. cost per procedure: $730 35% variation 333%	Interventional Diagnostics: Lab count, Imaging time (MRI), Imaging counts (X-ray)
	8% All Other Avg. cost per procedure: $1580 67% 155% variation	All Other: varies by service

$9,950	$8,270		$18,220
45% 162% variation	67% 184% variation	=	55% 155% variation

As described in the above figure, you'll see that the average direct lumbar spine fusion cost over 852 procedures is $9,950 or 54% per procedure. The average service center cost per procedure is $8,270 or 46%, for an average lumbar spine fusion cost of $18,220. Many of the direct costs such as supplies, blood and drugs are not as manageable as service center costs; however, there are opportunities for bulk discounts and supply rate negotiations.

The area of variability and opportunity lies within the service center costs. Could we improve efficiency in the number of OR case minutes by ensuring minimizing minutes that are not devoted to actual surgical time? Are efficiencies available for room-in to room-out time as well as staff time? Are the Admission, Discharge, and Transfer (ADT) processes being adhered to and being executed effectively? Are patient stays longer than clinically necessary? These are the service center costs that are manageable and if done so effectively, we can reduce the current cost variation that ranges from 55% – 155%. It's safe to say that many variations can be traced back to processes. Effective identification and management of process variation allows leaders to place emphasis on necessary factors that drive variation. Let's highlight four core process variation oversight techniques:

1. Gap Analysis/Risk and Workflow Assessment – At a minimum, conduct an operational assessment annually to track performance year over year. Use results to implement process improvement plans.

2. Data Gathering – This is a great opportunity to leverage technology for extracting key metrics in report formats that are necessary for analyzing the success and weaknesses of current processes to move toward service center goals.

3. Implement Standard Operating Procedures – All stakeholders should be informed, aware and accountable for service center success. Development and improvement of standard processes keeps everyone aware of target goals and how they are to be accomplished. This also sets the standard of expectation, so when dips occur, they may easily be identified and corrected. Standards also allow service centers to compare current, past and future status for measuring success.

Preventive Care Services

Implementing a preventive services protocol is an opportunity to move away from chronic disease management and acute care management to instead prioritize preventive service line management. We've described the services that CMS deems as preventive already in this book, but ask yourself if there are other services that can be provided to keep chronically ill patients in care and reduce risk of hospitalization or exacerbation of symptoms. An important component of preventive services and overall care management is patient engagement. Services on the periphery of preventive services such as chronic care management (CCM), principal care management (PCM) and transitional care management (TCM) offer a gateway into solidifying an evidence-based preventive care financial management program within an organization.

110

Transitional care is a major component of preventive care as we seek to prevent hospital readmissions post-discharge. A best practice strategy employed by hospital systems and community providers alike is a TCM protocol. Within this protocol, the hospital or facility prepares for a patient's discharge back into the community through communicating and transitioning to outpatient care.

Exhibit 3.12 Application of Transitional Care Management (TCM) into Preventive Services Protocols

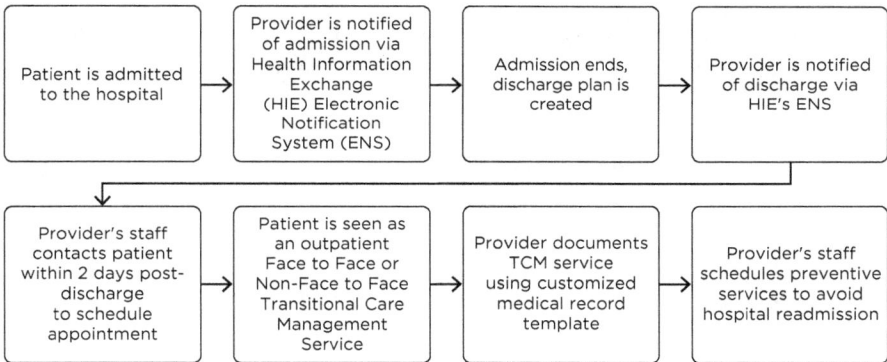

The above TCM protocol describes the pathway of care transition. In addition to the clear benefits to patient care and readmission reduction by keeping patients within an active care plan, there are financial opportunities that may be leveraged when implementing a TCM protocol. Rather than reporting the typical evaluation and management CPT codes for treatment after hospitalization, providers who meet the TCM CPT code requirements may report these services at a higher rate of reimbursement than a typical office visit CPT code.

Exhibit 3.13 Income Potential

CPT/HCPCS	Medicare Rate	Work RVU	Reimbursement Guidelines
99495	$241.22	2.78	Patient seen within 14 days of discharge, Moderate Medical Decision Making
99496	$324.79	3.79	Patient seen within 7 days of discharge, High Medical Decision Making

Data based on Novitas JL Solutions. District of Columbia (01) Locality.

Throughout this book, we've placed significant emphasis on leveraging concepts of value-based care to not only improve patient outcomes but to also improve revenue by financially aligning your organization with these innovative and complex reimbursement models. As federal, state and commercial payers are evolving payment strategies, there is the requirement for provider organizations to share in the financial risk of care delivery, thus explaining the slow demise of FFS reimbursement structures and the rapid progression of value-based reimbursement (VBR). This is a constant evolution that needs continuous monitoring and with regular internal financial re-modeling.

Several key factors to shared financial risk that are equally prioritized in a VBR model include:

- Payment for Quality not Quantity
- Encouraged Prevention
- Quadruple Aim and Care Collaboration

Pulling each of these components together requires the provider to utilize evidence-based practices to reduce costs or "share" with the payer in the financial downside "risk" of failure to produce expected outcomes. Shared financial risk requires the provider and the payer to sit in both the driver and passenger seats as they navigate to improved healthcare outcomes resulting in projected cost savings.

Technology Optimization for Service Line Improvement

Risk-based contracting for population health management is grounded in simple math. Healthcare organizations that exceed total medical spending targets for these contracts effectively absorb a penalty. Those that keep expenses below these targets create savings they can keep. With multiple at-risk contracts, Mass General Brigham currently is at risk for the costs of care for over 500,000 patients, making medical expense management critically important—especially for high-risk, high-utilization populations. A typical patient within the health system's integrated care programs, for example, is 76 years old, has more than three acute-care hospitalizations per year, and is taking more than 12 active medications.

At the same time, Mass General Brigham recognizes that it is inconsistent with provider values and workflow to manage different subpopulations of patients to different targets. Therefore, Mass General Brigham has created an Internal Performance Framework (IPF) that uses a single set of performance targets, Cost Standardized Medical Expenses (CSME), and a single incentive pool for all Mass General Brigham contracts, with the goal of promoting the best possible care for all patients while also meeting the demands of multiple external contract requirements. To gain insights into the populations, care teams needed the ability to organize and study a combination of data across the enterprise. In a parallel need, financial decision makers required insights into clinical performance.

To enable the analysis of current performance and drive clinical transformation, Mass General Brigham implemented a late-binding enterprise data warehouse platform (EDW) from Health Catalyst. The EDW aggregates clinical, financial, operational, claims, and other data to create consistent views of the data to inform decisions for providers and managers alike. It uses common patient/provider identifiers to assure accurate identification of both patients and providers. This in turn supports the use of flags to easily identify high-risk patient cohorts.

The ACO/shared risk management and population health advanced analytics gives Mass General Brigham new insight to manage populations with superior care and minimum waste. It measures and tracks the expenses and utilization that drive population trends associated with risk contracts, and identifies patient populations that generate higher expenses.[23]

What can we learn from Mass General?

1. Determine the risk-reward of entering into risk-based contracts

2. Understand your internal capabilities of meeting expectations of such an arrangement

3. Re-engineer company culture, best practices, technology and workflow improvements to meet risk-based contract requirements

4. Measure performance and recalibrate when and where needed

Service Enhancers

Each healthcare organization has an area of specialty, board certification and population need. We prioritize the services provided by leveraging our skills, licensure and the needs of our communities. These baseline healthcare services are maximized by enhancing them with additional services that complement the original service offerings. For example, an organization that performs in-office physical examinations may collaborate with a local laboratory for in-suite laboratory services. This type of service enhancer is for the benefit and convenience of the patient. In this type of arrangement, the original healthcare facility may not profit from these non-billable laboratory services. However, no additional salaries or equipment are necessary as those are covered by the laboratory.

Service enhancers that may positively impact revenue would require additional monitoring or testing for a patient population that could benefit from billable services. Examples would include remote patient monitoring or other diagnostic testing and monitoring. The pathway to optimizing service enhancers is to follow standard of care, improving patient outcomes, medical record documentation, and leveraging billable opportunities. In the RPM example, the facility is adding a new billable service to the existing care plan that not only adds value to the clinician by monitoring a potential chronic illness during times that the patient is not in the office receiving face-to-face care, but this service is an enhancement both clinically and financially to the original service.

Another key component of optimizing service enhancers is understanding your current and future patient population's needs and access to resources like technology and at-home medical devices. Patients with chronic illnesses are typically good candidates for service enhancers as they may require additional support in between appointments. Continuous engagement with chronically ill patients mitigates risks of illness exacerbation through monitoring and regular communication intervals. Those patients who may be challenged with Social Determinants of Health (SDOH) may lack the technology to support external monitoring and testing. There are however, local, state, federal and even commercial insurance resources to assist individuals in securing the care options.

Virtual Care Delivery and Remote Patient Monitoring

As telehealth becomes more standard as a care delivery method, it becomes time to focus on applying strategic planning to ensure long-term viability. Developing a sustainable telehealth model includes outlining the regulations that will impact your organization in the future and developing a strategic plan to address future needs.

Telehealth service waivers that are temporary will require a long-term sustainability approach. A few of the key tenets of 1135 Waiver – Public Health Emergency (PHE) include:[24]

- Removal of geographic restrictions for mental health telehealth services by allowing patient's home to be originating site
- In-person visit requirements for mental/behavioral health services
- Continuation of reimbursing audio-only visits
- Reduction of beneficiary coinsurance for colorectal CA screenings that result in diagnostic tests
- Electronic Prescribing for Controlled Substances (EPCS) mandate
- Opioid Treatment Program (OTP) use of audio-only to furnish counseling & therapy services using a CPT/HCPCS modifier
- Clinical laboratory specimen collection and travel allowance

As of this writing, the COVID-19 public health emergency was set to end on May 11, 2023.[25] Prior to that date, healthcare organizations had to reconcile how to best incorporate the tenets of 1135 Waiver into their organizations. Our recommended approach is to focus on internal opportunities. Two major categories of the PHE were the expansion of telehealth services and reduction of obstacles to care resulting from administrative burdens. We needed to to understand the waivers and how those waivers impacted operations. This also required steadfast review of each year's CMS Final Rule located within the Federal Register.

While incorporating service enhancers into organizational modeling, consider the following strategies to incorporate the Current Year CMS Final Rule, create an internal sustainability measure, and implement KPIs to measure success.

Exhibit 3.14 Leveraging the CMS Final Rule to Create a Sustainable Hybrid Telehealth Model

CMS 2023 Rule	Sustainability Measure	KPIs
Conversion Factor Reduction	Analyze fee schedule and compare payer reimbursement	Major payers are paying 150% of Medicare
Removal of Geographic Restrictions	Incorporate Incident-To billing for telehealth services	Run CPT Reports
Physician Assistant's to Bill Medicare Directly	Hire 3 PA's and prepare to bill while physicians are rounding at hospitals	Staffing ratio analysis
EPCS Mandate Enforcement	Review EMR settings for EPCS set up	Track number of CDS ePrescribing
Reimbursement Expiration with the PHE	Track service codes that expire when the Public Health Emergency expires	Run CPT Reports

We have unique overlapping priorities which allow us to essentially, "kill a few birds with one stone." As we pull together clinical and service line data for virtual care delivery, we can also use this data for successful value-based payment program participation. If your organization decides to use a stand-alone telehealth platform for documentation, consider the transferability of that data back to your EMR. Some

Chapter 3: Financial Planning

platforms only allow for PDF upload of medical notes. This data format may not meet MIPS and other value-based program reporting measures. The data must be in the appropriate format and aligned with the correct software fields such as structured data formats for tracking and reporting MIPS and other program measures.

Promoting Interoperability is one of the MIPS and Advanced Alternative Payment Program measures. Reporting period 2022 ushered in a new mandate entitled, "Safety Assurance Factors for EHR Resilience (SAFER)." The SAFER mandate is for covered entities to conduct an EMR self-assessment to optimize safety and workforce optimization of an organizational EMR. The SAFER self-assessment is a mandate that is in addition to, and does not replace, the Security Risk Assessment (SRA) requirement which will continue to be scored.

The Office of National Coordinator (ONC) deems the SAFER assessment as a critical component to ensure the proper long-term use of EMRs nationwide for sustainable healthcare delivery.

Combination of In-Person Care Delivery and Virtual Care Delivery

The industry has been forced to adopt telehealth and hybrid business models during a time of unprecedented change. In order to sustain these changes, we want to leverage strategies for long-term incorporation of best practices for both virtual and in-person care delivery to deploy sustainable hybrid care. As we consider service-line optimization, we want to understand our patient population and their specific needs, expectations, and norms.

Below is an illustration of patient telehealth usage over a specific period of time during the recent PHE based on factors including age, gender, sexual orientation, ethnicity, and physical ability. Utilizing the below consumer trends in accessing telehealth services creates understanding of the telehealth utilization patterns of our patient population based on factors that allow us to customize our engagement to fit individual population needs.

117

Exhibit 3.15 Telemedicine Use in the Last Four Weeks

National Estimate	June 29, 2022 – July 11, 2022	June 23, 2021 – July 5, 2021
United States	22.8%	24.5%
18 – 29 years old	19.2%	22.5%
40 – 49 years old	22.6%	23.6%
60 – 69 years old	23.9%	25.1%
70 – 79 years old	27.0%	26.6%
Male	20.4%	21.5%
Female	25.2%	27.2%
Gay or Lesbian	25.3%	No Data
Transgender	27.4%	No Data
Hispanic or Latino	23.0%	27.6%
White	21.5%	22.6%
Black	28.0%	30%
Asian	25.4%	24.8%
Disabled	32.9%	38.8%

CDC Statistics[26]

This is the type of data we want to take into consideration as we customize service lines for individuals within our communities to improve population health. This data gives us opportunities to engage with specific patient populations based on trends. Messaging and engagement strategies are customized based on the population we are attempting to reach. Inclusion and diversity based on our understanding of our patient base can occur by getting in touch with our audience using messaging that speaks directly to each unique population. Utilizing the above CDC telehealth statistics, we learn that a considerable number of disabled patients seek telehealth services. Our engagement should connect us to that audience.

Avoiding Poor Care Outcomes with Hybrid Care Delivery

It's evident that concerns about viral disease exposure directly influence patients to stay away from medical facilities, which in turn negatively impacts population health. When patients aren't getting their screenings, emerging conditions can go unnoticed. Additionally, patients may be getting sicker because they aren't managing their chronic conditions as well as they could with the guidance of a healthcare professional. For patients who suffer from one or more chronic illnesses, exacerbation of these diseases will occur when not monitored closely. One way to keep patients healthy is to identify health risks as soon as possible, provide treatment, and document illness severity to the highest level so that we report the acuity of our patient population. This allows for the appropriate rate setting and reimbursement of a particular population.

Healthcare organizations' margins are already razor thin, so we want to ensure that necessary service lines are identified, implemented and managed in a manner that provides a long-term positive impact on illness outcomes, which in turn improves revenue potential. Service line analysis areas should include:

- Exacerbation of chronic illness – Determine if patients could benefit from RPM tracking
- Untreated acute illnesses – Investigate trends in acute illnesses that have the potential to lead to hospitalization or pre-chronic illnesses
- Missed screenings – Manage cancellations and no-shows to recall patients as well as prioritize the importance of screening procedures and testing
- Unmonitored bloodwork – Collection, review, communication and action on all lab work especially those with abnormal limits
- Reduction in elective procedures – Identify standard of care and medical necessity for elective procedures that may improve quality of life and daily acts of living
- Decreased in-person visits – Trends in shifts of service location provide an opportunity to expand virtual care delivery options
- Patients transition from commercial insurance to Medicaid – Consumer job loss or transitions may impact benefits options thereby altering a healthcare organization's payer mix
- Workforce Burnout – Retention and recruiting may impact capacity to maintain patient volumes and services

- Hospital Readmissions – Avoid readmissions by implementing a transition of care program that includes collaborative discharge planning

Telehealth Utilization Best Practices

Organizations are looking for the best ways to incorporate best practices for both in-person and virtual visits. Although the COVID-19 Public Health Emergency has ended and many waivers will follow, telehealth delivery in some capacity is going to be necessary. These changes will impact the current payment parity for telehealth services. There are service types that are best provided in person; however, there are many services that could be offered and successfully managed in a hybrid delivery model. The key is to determine the factors that will impact a hybrid telehealth model. We can achieve optimal telehealth utilization by taking into consideration the following care and patient engagement strategies:

These include:

- Prioritizing chronic care management
- Addressing co-morbidities
- Increasing access to mental health services
- Focusing on interoperability and data sharing
- Improving User Experience via patient portal

Our long-term workflows and service line management should take into consideration the unique factors of in-office vs telehealth care delivery. A few of these factors would include:

- Identifying organizational needs based on the visit type and prepare in advance
- Optimizing technology for both in-person and telehealth visits
- Reducing virus spread
- Enforcing patient and workforce safety
- Bolstering patient engagement
- Optimizing technology

Exhibit 3.16 Below are a few considerations for comparing in-person care vs virtual care:

In Person Care	Telehealth / Virtual Care
In-person waiting room Physical waiting will include wait times for form completion and delays resulting from other patients' appointments.	Virtual waiting room Determine what messaging is available while patients wait virtually. Consider the ability for patients to complete eForms.
PPE and Social Distancing Management of mask usage to mitigate the threat of virus spread.	Remote encounter excludes infection risks. Patients who may be immunocompromised may feel safer avoiding contact with others.
Office/exam room overhead Determine expenses related to in-person care delivery location expenses.	Reduced Overhead It may appear that overhead expenses may be reduced; however, this isn't always the case.
In-Person TOS collections Face-to-face consumer interaction would allow for increased time of service collection of copayments, overdue balances and coinsurances.	Touchless payment options Opportunities exist to improve payment options to mirror those that patients are familiar with utilizing in other areas of daily living.

We want to comfort and educate the consumers who are still wary about receiving care virtually through the lens of our unique patients' perspectives. We can minimize their concerns by educating patients about the effectiveness of telehealth services. Informing patients about your organization's security measures will put them at ease. Offering general insurance benefit information adds credibility to telehealth services – if their insurance covers it, there must be something valuable. Use your organization's website and social media to dispel myths and offer credible information. As patients are waiting in either a virtual or in-person waiting room, use that time for education – display posters or pre-record looping information regarding telehealth and in-person care. Patients are busy, so making sure they receive appointment reminders in intervals leading up to their appointment will increase the likelihood that they will keep an appointment.

The flip side to this is prioritizing post-telehealth visit follow-up, because "out of sight out of mind" could build barriers to care. For face-to-face visits, we have the patient in front of us which allows us to review orders, provide prescriptions, make follow-up appointments, coordinate external testing and referrals and make a final attempt to collect owed monies. These functions are challenged during telehealth visits, as after the patient visit, the healthcare provider disconnects the appointment leaving minimal staff follow-up with the patient. Follow up with patients before and after telehealth visits to avoid "out of sight out of mind." We want to keep patients in care by developing virtual check-out processes and by creating wellness campaigns that provide education on chronic illness management.

Below are a few tactics to prioritize patient engagement to increase care plan adherence and decrease illness exacerbation:

- Pre-visit and post-visit survey or follow-up communication
- Direct patient-to-provider bios and profiles via practice website
- Offer telehealth visit instructions
- Update website PHE safety protocols
- Provide links on health & insurance literacy
- Offer secure online touchless payments
- Publish the organization's financial policy on a secure patient portal
- Advertise use of your patient portal via social media and practice website
- Leverage eStatements via patient portal
- Offer electronic balance reminders via patient portal

Our patients are living in a touchless environment outside of healthcare. Let's incorporate this technology into our patient engagement strategies.

Payment Parity

Providers are benefiting from the CMS waiver authorizing telehealth services to be paid at the same rate as office visit reimbursements. It's not surprising that overutilization of telehealth services could have a downstream impact on physician reimbursement as insurance companies attempt to ensure they are paying for the same level of effort, complexity and medical decision-making for telehealth vs. in-office care.

It's common for commercial payers to follow Medicare's reimbursement guidelines and within the PHE this is no exception. Many but not all payers are following Medicare's lead. In order to eliminate gaps in reimbursement, we want to stay in touch with our commercial payers on a regular basis to see when telehealth reimbursement waivers end and to identify changes to previous telehealth policies. Commercial payers' policies on reimbursing audio only visits should also be investigated if that is a mode of service delivery your organization is utilizing.

With the use of telehealth service delivery, there can be the tendency to exclude discussions on Social Determinants of Health (SDoH) during virtual visits. Patients who are in our care virtually, however, may continue to struggle with socioeconomic, environmental and other factors that impact their health. There are ICD-10-CM codes ranging from Z55 to Z65 to report a patient's SDOH. These codes allow for demonstrating complexity while also customizing future telehealth service needs based on tracking and trending SDOH ICD-10-CM code utilization.

As payers are relying on utilization review protocols, providers should ensure that documentation of telehealth visits demonstrates the same effort and risk to morbidity and mortality as if that visit were conducted at the office in person. It's more important than ever to ensure specificity in diagnosis coding and prioritizing Hierarchical Condition Categories (HCCs) to demonstrate risk scores. It's more important than ever to demonstrate complexity with diagnosis-specificity to justify E/M levels.

Clinical Documentation Improvement

Most if not all healthcare funding sources rely on clinical documentation to understand and pay for healthcare expenses for specific beneficiary populations. These funding sources utilize healthcare providers' clinical documentation and ICD-10-CM (diagnosis code) selection to apply risk factors to populations. These risk factors are adjusted using a score that is based on a number of factors that include geography, age, and risk of mortality and morbidity. Healthcare providers who fail to demonstrate accurate health risks and complexity for chronically ill patient populations are in fact describing an inaccurate description of a patient's risk. By doing so, the entities who rely on risk calculation will inaccurately calculate healthcare costs and payments for the impacted patient population. These inaccurate calculations have a negative downstream effect on the overall healthcare ecosystem. One of the negative impacts to the healthcare provider is decreased reimbursement based on the inaccurately demonstrated risk. The entities who regularly utilize risk adjustment for healthcare funding include those entities that may in some way reimburse healthcare providers either using a shared-risk model or federal and state programs. As risk sharing continues to result in cost savings and improved outcomes, expect to see the entities that utilize risk adjustment continue to expand.

Exhibit 3.17 Key Entities That Use Risk Adjustment

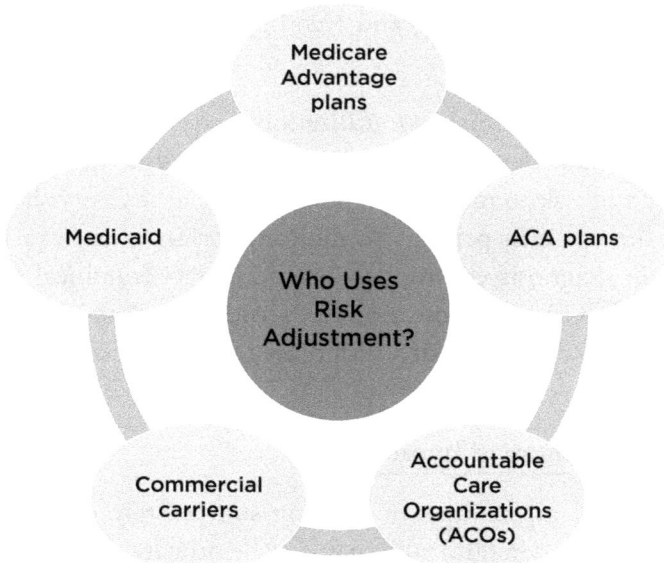

Clinical Documentation Improvement (CDI) does minimize inclusion of unspecified codes unless a specific code cannot be applied. It also justifies illness severity and risk of mortality while following medical decision making (MDM) guidelines and provides an accurate depiction of healthcare costs.

We can incorporate CDI into reimbursement strategies by utilizing SDOH, remaining vigilant, and staying on the lookout for payer contract amendments. It's also important to closely monitor commercial payer adjustment codes and denial trends. Including a monthly review of online commercial payer reimbursement guidelines allows us to determine any changes to telehealth reimbursement by payer. One strategy of managing commercial payer telehealth reimbursement guidelines is to create and update a reimbursement matrix. Keep in mind that commercial payers have unique guidelines that *will* change and will not be easy to locate, which is why the development of your own matrix of rules is essential.

Exhibit 3.18 Sample Payor Telehealth Reimbursement Guidelines Matrix

Payer	Telehealth CPT Codes	Payer Link
Utilize your organization's payer participation list to extract those payers to which your organization submits claims on a regular basis.	Many services that are listed in your fee schedule may be approved to be conducted and paid via telehealth. Extract the most commonly used CPT/HCPCS codes from your charge description master (CDM) as well as the payer's fee schedules.	Document each payer's website section that outlines telehealth payment guidelines. This may require some digging as some payers embed this information in website sections that may not be easily accessible. Check for updates at least quarterly and notify organizational stakeholders of updates.

CMS implemented several Medicare telehealth billing guidelines for medical group practices during the COVID-19 public health emergency (PHE). This is a downloadable CMS resource that outlines Medicare Telehealth Services payment guidelines. This matrix is updated by CMS and may be included in your internal telehealth reimbursement matrix. As CMS sets the tone for most reimbursement rules, staying up to date on and comparing CMS' telehealth payment guidelines to commercial payers is ideal.

Exhibit 3.19 List of Medicare Telehealth Services[27]

List of Medicare Telehealth Services Effective January 1, 2023 – Updated November 1, 2022				
Code	Short Descriptor	Status	Can Audio-only Interaction Meet the Requirement	Medicare Payment Limitations
Approved CPT/ HCPCS Code	Brief description of CPT/ HCPCS Code	Guidance on when payment approval ends (e.g., Available through 12/31/23 or Temporary Addition for the PHE; Expires with PHE plus 151 days)	Yes or No guidance on whether or not CPT/HCPCS Code can be provided as an Audio-only encounter	Guidance on limitation on payments for CPT/ HCPCS Code to include: Bundled code, non-covered service or statutory exclusion

As part of telehealth service line management, it's important to check state guidelines which may supersede federal telehealth mandates. Documentation for all telehealth services must indicate that services rendered were performed via a telehealth method. Telehealth service documentation requirements for E/M visits 99201–99215 must meet the criteria established by CPT guidelines. Patient consent for telehealth services must be obtained verbally or in written form. We must also document the type of technology being used. If a code is time-based, evidence of time must be documented. It's also required that we document any other persons present during a telehealth visit. If exchanged asynchronously, videos, images and communications must be stored and retained according to state regulation. CMS has a full list of telehealth documentation guidelines that may be included in an organizational telehealth delivery and documentation protocol.

As we prioritize documentation of visits, we also want to prioritize patient communication, education and engagement. An informed patient is a compliant patient. Keeping patients in care starts with consistent communication. Avoid non-adherence to care plans by optimizing the use of a patient portal to remind patients of healthcare milestones and necessary testing orders. By addressing acute problems via telehealth, we prevent exacerbation of chronic illnesses, which decreases health-care costs and increases our Value-Based Payment scores. We may also enhance consumer health literacy by including them in monitoring their chronic illnesses virtually through:

- At-Home Medical Devices
- Visit Summaries
- Virtual visit check-out process
- Wearable Technology
- Remote Patient Monitoring

Remote Physiologic Monitoring (RPM) Treatment Management Services

Remote physiologic monitoring (RPM) is a unique care management function that allows physicians and other qualified healthcare professionals and clinical staff to obtain and monitor physiological results from devices at the patient's home to manage specific treatment plans. The devices used must be defined by the FDA and ordered by a qualified healthcare professional or physician. RPM is a "monitoring" technique used in conjunction with an established care plan that eliminates the opportunity for billing RPM for time that can be reported for other monitoring services. Since RPM is an extension of care management, it may be reported during the same service period as other care management services such as:

- Chronic care management services (99437, 99439, 99487, 99489, 99490, 99491)
- Principal care management services (99424, 99425, 99426, 99427)
- Transitional care management services (99495, 99496)
- Behavioral health integration services (99484, 99492, 99493, 99494)

Please note that CPT/HCPCS codes are updated annually so it is wise to check your CPT/HCPCS manual to ensure the codes listed remain applicable. RPM is a popular service as providers are expanding virtual care delivery and the need to monitor patients virtually. Since it may only be reported once per calendar month, we want to ensure that we have the ability to capture all device data for the specific treatment plan and billing. As RPM is connected to a treatment plan, it may not be billed on the same date of service as the Evaluation and Management code series 99211–99205. Remote Physiological Monitoring will include synchronous provider/patient communication. Again, CPT codes are updated annually, however; RPM codes may include the following:[28]

CPT Code	Description	Washington, DC Rate
99453	Rem mntr physiol param setup	$23.46
99454	Rem mntr physiol param dev	$60.89
99457	Rem mntr physiol 1st 20 min	$56.00
99458	Rem mntr physiol ea addl 20 min	$44.89

Strategic Planning for RPM Implementation

Now that we've detailed RPM, let's examine its application into organizational service-line delivery. RPM can be beneficial for both provider and patient communications. As you consider either implementing or optimizing RPM into your organization, ask yourself these questions:

1. Are internal and patient-facing technology needs met?
2. How will troubleshooting be managed?
3. Are EMR/PM CPT codes correct?
4. What are the results of a financial analysis?
5. What are the results of care plan improvement analysis?
6. Is there an RPM note template available for documentation?
7. Is RPM data generated using structured data?
8. Are there payer-specific reimbursement guidelines that need to be met?
9. Have payer denial or non-payment trends been uncovered?
10. How are patients adjusting to out-of-pocket RPM expenses?

We can leverage the MGMA Body of Knowledge (BOK) to create sustainable hybrid telehealth and face-to-face care delivery models by focusing our efforts on each domain, creating measures that you want to meet based on your unique organizational needs and establishing achievable benchmarks to gauge your success or improvement needs. Below is an example of using the BOK domains to create sustainability measures for a hybrid telehealth delivery model.

Exhibit 3.20 Example of Leveraging the BOK for Hybrid Care Delivery Sustainability

BOK Domain	Sustainability Measure	KPIs
Operations Management	Optimization of telehealth technology	30% increase of virtual visits
Financial Management	Interpreting and applying new E & M guidelines	Increased use of 99214
Human Resource Management	Remote workforce monitoring and compliance	50% increased staff turnover
Risk & Compliance Management	Workforce and patient safety from COVID-19 exposure	No new provider COVID-19 infections
Organizational Governance	Reconstruction of cash flow projections	$5K increase in PPE expenses
Transformative Healthcare Delivery	Redefine patient care flows to include telehealth services	Automation of all intake forms

MGMA® Body of Knowledge

3.6 Critical Policies for Theft Deterrence and Revenue Protection

Theft in medical practices, particularly embezzlement, has been around for a long time and unfortunately, much like the cost of supplies during the pandemic, the rate of theft seems to be rising. The amounts are increasing and the tactics are becoming more complex. In December 2021, an employee at an Indiana medical practice was sentenced for stealing over $270,000 over five years by falsifying books, sending additional payroll checks to himself, and more. In April 2022, a woman was charged in Australia for stealing over $565,000 from her employer through the use of the employer's credit card and bank account over the course of a decade. In May 2022, a woman in Florida pleaded no contest to scheming and defrauding more than $283,000 from her place of work by writing herself checks.. These three examples alone comprise over a million dollars in revenue that was siphoned away from medical practices.

Where Theft Happens

Theft that takes place in the medical practice is most often a crime of opportunity, meaning the proper protocols and steps required to minimize theft have not been implemented. There are many methods of theft from practices and they range in complexity with the easier opportunities taking place much more frequently than others.

Frequently Seen

- Stealing of cash payments that come across the front desk or into the billing department
- Misuse/abuse of company credit cards or bank accounts
- Lying about timesheets
- Stealing supplies
- Theft of petty cash

More Complex

- Falsifying employee records to obtain payroll for a non-existent employee
- Submitting false invoices to fake vendors and paying the invoices out
- Changing the EFT information to personal bank accounts
- Taking virtual credit cards home and processing personally
- Setting up third-party merchant accounts to run patient cards through
- Posting refunds for overpayments and pocketing the rebate check

Prevention Methods

In each of the examples listed above, it is evident that a few things take place:

- Minimal oversight
- Too few or too many hands on the money
- Failure to audit and reconcile

All of these fall under areas of process control. To help deter theft, you need to make it as hard as possible for someone to steal from the practice and get away with it. Here are some areas to strengthen to reduce the possibility of theft:

1. Hiring Practices – Implement background checks for employees and actually verify references that are requested and received

2. Human Resources – Develop policies with stern consequences for theft including all types of theft listed above

3. Minimize Cash – Minimize the use of cash at the front desk by offering several methods of payment and all forms of credit card or cash transfer apps (ex. PayPal).

4. Secure Credit Card Information – Do not store the full credit card number for patients in a way that is visible for staff. Once a credit card number has been entered all but the last four digits should be hidden.

5. Reduce Virtual Credit Cards – These types of payments slowly chip away at revenue anyway. Opt out of virtual credit card payments whenever possible.

6. TOS Reconciliations – Everyone who takes money for time-of-service payments should have to document transactions received on a daily basis. In an ideal situation, end users would collect money from the patient and post it in the practice management system. At the end of their shift, they should print the day's total and validate that the total cash and credit card receipts match the printout. They should then initial and seal the money, receipts and report in a lock bag for the manager to deposit.

7. Ledger to PM System Reconciliations

   a. On a daily basis, evaluate deposits received in the bank to confirm that cash deposits documented made it to the bank in full.

      i. The total being verified should match the total amount of TOS collections pulled from the lock bags in addition to any checks received from payers.

   b. On a weekly basis, review EFTs posted to the practice management system against deposits to the bank account and confirm receipt.

   c. On a monthly basis, balance the general ledger to the monthly bank statement and monthly deposits received in the PM system.

      i. For deposits in the general ledger that are not in the PM system, notify the billing manager to ensure timely posting

      ii. For deposits in the PM system that are not in the general ledger, review the payer's remittance for payment information and identify where the missing payment has gone

      iii. For deposits in the bank account that are not in the general ledger, notify the billing manager to ensure timely posting

      iv. For deposits in the general ledger that are not in the bank account, evaluate the days and times of prospective deposits, confirm they are not duplicates, and refer back to the daily TOS reports from staff

   d. Logging staff activity documenting TOS collections in the PM system has the added bonus of date/time/user-stamping the transaction. In addition, the practice should keep a log of deposits headed to the bank along with information about the total deposit amount and the employee taking the deposit to the bank.

8. Auditing: Invest in a third-party bookkeeper and medical billing auditing company to perform audits at least annually

9. Spread the work: If only one individual is responsible for payment collections, posting, and reconciliation, they have a lot of power with which to hide theft.

The best strategy for workplace theft deterrence is to implement strong processes for oversight and auditing. Assuming your staff is trustworthy or would never fall on hard times is a bad idea. Even the kindest, most loyal employees have stolen from companies with "the intent to pay back" before it got out of hand.

3.7 Dashboard Best Practices for Optimized Financial Review

Data is powerful. It's even more powerful when it can be used to improve the metrics of the trends within the areas that it is visualizing to the beholder of that information. The "out of the box" dashboards that are accessible in most software platforms are those that are fed information via structured data. That structured data is populated into the respective dashboard fields to visualize the data elements extracted from primary source information. Dashboard data is certainly a bad data in, bad data out scenario.

The importance of accurate information populating into a dashboard cannot be understated. Those who rely on dashboard information rely on the data being received and populated to be accurate. An example of dashboard data that is used to make important decisions would be Merit-based Incentive Payment System (MIPS). Data from the reportable quality measures are extracted from various sections of the medical record and populate into a dashboard. This type of out-of the box dashboard may leave little room for customization; however, if all program reporting details are available, little customization may be necessary.

Let's consider financial dashboards that are customizable based on varying KPIs within your organization. KPIs are the critical (key) indicators of progress toward an intended result. KPIs provide a focus for strategic and operational improvement, create an analytical basis for decision making and help focus attention on what matters most. According to Becker's Hospital Review, "Key Performance Indicators (KPIs) are defined as metrics used to measure key business processes and reflect strategic performance."[29] Or, as Peter Drucker famously said, "What gets measured gets managed."

Inclusion of KPIs in customizable financial dashboards allows one to track multiple metrics simultaneously, across varying departments, cost centers, and strategic opportunities. The most effective way of leveraging dashboards is to customize relevant metrics, each providing a unique outlook of a whole picture. Within the below dashboard we are able to track multiple KPIs simultaneously.

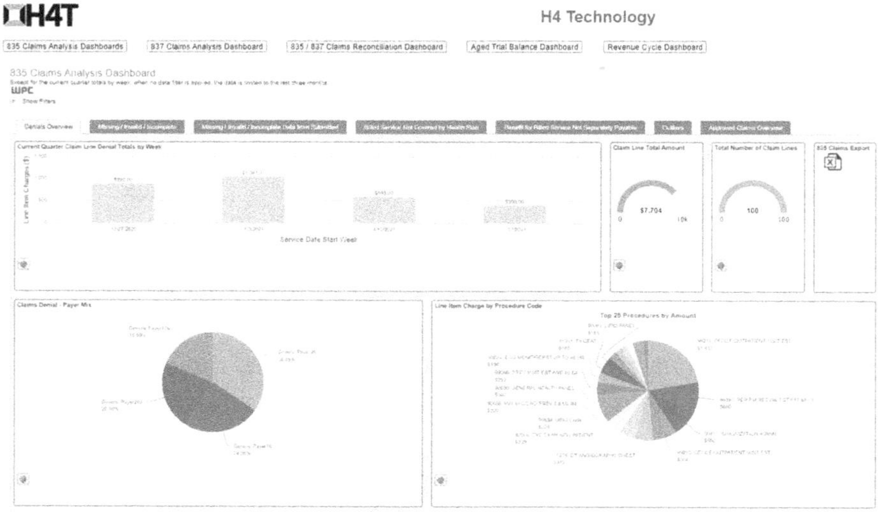

Exhibit 3.21 H4 Technology Claims Analysis Dashboard[30]

By analyzing the above dashboard, one may use these data elements for the following purposes:

1. Dollar amount and age of denial types – Create worklists for staff to perform Accounts Receivable follow-up

2. Reason for denials – Improve workflows, training and claim scrubbing to prevent future denials

3. Number of claim lines – Allows for tracking and correction of code sequencing as well as proper modifier usage

4. Denial percentage by payer type – Uncovers compliance or lack thereof for respective payer reimbursement guidelines

5. CPT/HCPCS denial type by payer – Uncovers coding inaccuracies that require corrective action

There could certainly be other uses for the above metrics; however, there are certain corrective actions that may be taken based on best practice and organizational needs. It's up to the user to decide how to use this information. Visually analyzing dashboards using KPIs improves one's ability to track areas of opportunity to pivot as necessary. Dashboards are also helpful in breaking down high-level summaries to granular details in just a few clicks. Include key organizational factors to review within your dashboard.

The below management dashboard eliminates the need (unless it's necessary) to run multiple reports independently. Accessing multiple forms of data provides a birds eye view so that one may manage the effectiveness of others. Dashboard management is an efficient way of managing a remote workforce using various metrics that several individuals are responsible for performing on a daily basis. Dashboards allow you to drill down to the specific details within each filtered metric. Having permission-based dashboards allows you to decide which users have access to various levels of data. Here is an example of a useful dashboard to track claims processing, aging balances, staff productivity and denials.

Dashboard customization using relevant or "key" performance indicators drives success in workflow improvement, compliance and meeting financial goals.

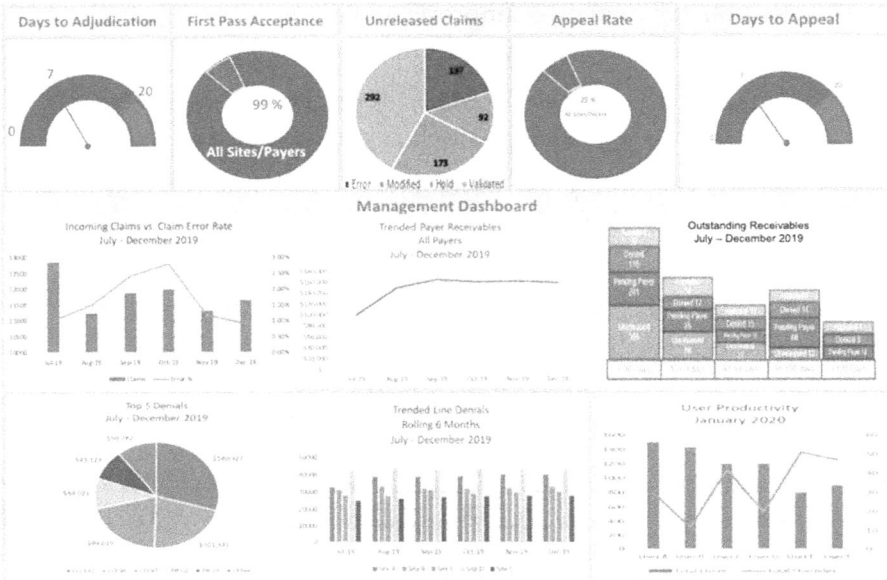

Exhibit 3.22 Ability Network/Inovalon Dashboard Management Tool

Metric Selection

Before we can measure, we have to decide *wha*t metric or data point to measure, which means we need to do some research. We have to identify which metrics are important for us to measure, why we want to measure it, and the goal of measuring that data. Only then can we work on defining and establishing the metrics that are going to work the best for our individual organizations.

When we select data, there is background regarding the metric selection. The "what" in the metric selection is going to be relevant to a financial or operational metric based on the data element we want to measure. The reason why we choose to measure a specific data element will most likely be based on historical performance or future projection needs. Integration of goals is critical to definition and metric selection.

We want to define the metrics that are relevant and important to our financial operations. We then want to outline and analyze key business processes. This will allow us to enhance decision making and lead

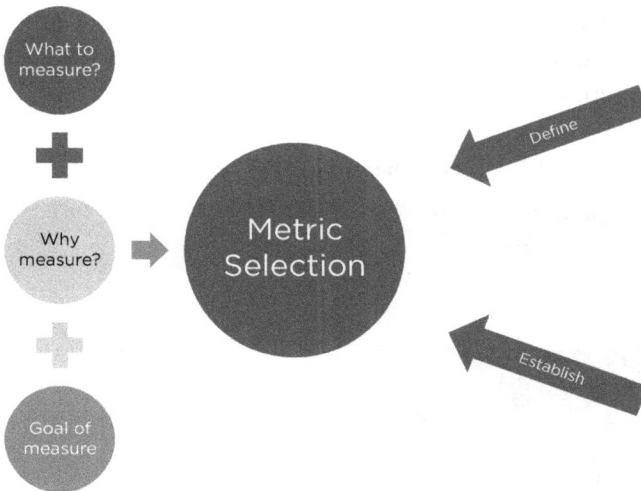

Exhibit 3.23 Metric Selection

toward pathways of financial success. We then use all of this information to take action – some responses might require immediate corrective actions, others will direct future strategic plans.

Metric selection and utilization allow us to measure achievement and adherence to business process goals. Good metrics provide objective evidence of progress toward achieving a desired result. They also measure what is intended to be measured to help inform better decision making and offer a comparison that gauges the degree of performance change over time.

It's important to note that oftentimes we use the terms KPIs and metrics interchangeably. KPIs are "key" or important metrics/data points that impact success or failure. We prioritize key performance indicators or key metrics, as they allow us to justify and quantify success with real data rather than hypotheses. Metrics that provide basic information that are not "key" to success are not usually measured. We prioritize key performance indicators (KPIs)/key metrics such as aging accounts receivable because it helps us measure performance. Metrics that aren't helpful in measuring performance might be useful but they are not "key."

Fluidity of metric selection and usage are critical to evolving healthcare operational, clinical and financial operations. Do not feel obligated to continue reporting for previously selected metrics.

Exhibit 3.24 MGMA Stat Poll: Changing KPIs

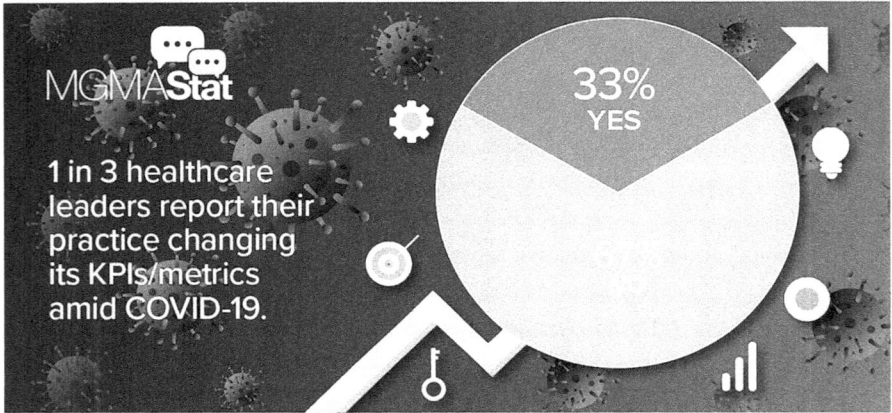

MGMA *Stat* poll. August 18, 2020 | Is your practice changing its KPIs/metrics amid COVID-19? | 472 responses. MGMA.COM/STAT, #MGMASTAT

Within the above MGMA poll, "Many respondents who indicated changes in KPIs and metrics noted a focus on tracking telehealth and phone visits. Other respondents mentioned updates for productivity, frequency (tracking measures weekly instead of monthly or annually) and care gaps. Amid COVID-19, savvy practices are changing what they measure and how often they measure key metrics, as normal business routines have changed dramatically."[31]

As the landscape evolves, the need to identify and track new or expanded metrics becomes more relevant. During the COVID-19 Public Health Emergency (PHE), metrics such as infection rates, volume of canceled elective procedures and dropped communications via telehealth were priorities for monitoring. As healthcare organizations' goals, needs and standards shift, find comfort in resetting previously necessary metrics based on current or future needs.

Key Performance Indicator (KPI) Curation

We've discussed the "key" in "key performance indicators." The "indicator" means that the information you have at hand isn't final or full but can help inform efficient decision-making. "KPIs can also help course-correct because they give a glimpse into the future,"[32] says Gabriel Tupula, CEO at Big Bang. The goal is to develop and curate meaningful KPIs that we understand should and will change over time, but provide us with much needed information about certain time periods that allow us to predict and prepare. When developing meaningful KPIs, we want to consider not only how the data will be used, but also who will use the data and the relevance to those stakeholders. When considering KPIs, it's wise to design them in a meaningful way that will allow KPIs to translate data in a meaningful manner.

Questions to answer when designing KPIs

- What questions regarding data do you get asked the most by stakeholders?
- What matters most to your audience?
- What's the main topic of discussion in meetings?
- Is the data currently being presented digestible by stakeholders?
- What decisions will be made with the data being presented?
- What are related internal and external forces impacting data?

Depending on the type of KPI you are using, the data revealed will shed light on vertical and horizontal trends. Vertical trends are those that are increasing or decreasing up or down. Horizontal KPIs are those that have parallel trends and allow us to view data over time.

There are several methods available when curating KPIs. One measurement strategy, after you've identified the metrics you want to measure, would be to review that data vertically as well as horizontally.

In the above table, KPIs are demonstrated vertically and horizontally. Analyzing KPIs in various formats allows us to see data in meaningful

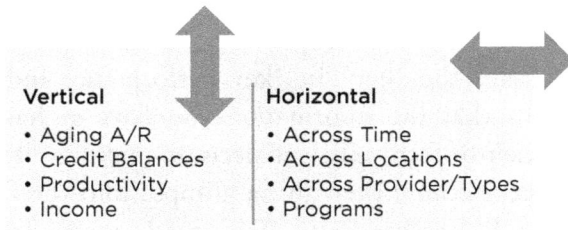

Vertical
- Aging A/R
- Credit Balances
- Productivity
- Income

Horizontal
- Across Time
- Across Locations
- Across Provider/Types
- Programs

Exhibit 3.25 KPI Curation Paths

ways to identify trends that are useful in decision making. Vertical KPIs that are trending data upward or downward allow one to measure success based on charting specific metrics. The goal for Accounts Receivable (A/R) would be for it to trend downward in aging – the higher the A/R, the longer on average it takes for payments to come in. Similarly, for credit balances, the fewer credit balances on patient accounts, the more accurate summation of total aging accounts receivables. Similarly to aging A/R and credit balances, productivity and income are two vertical KPIs. The difference with these two trends is the goal for them to move upward to demonstrate success. In most cases, higher productivity equates to higher income.

Horizontal KPIs such as data viewed "across" allows trending to be captured and measured in a manner in which the viewer may consider data that could be improved in parallel to others. For example, tracking data over periods of time allows one to determine successful days, months, quarters and years. This information could also be drilled down further to create a full picture of why parallel data may have changed, such as flu season creating an increased demand in sick visits or summertime reducing demand due to vacations. Determining the best way to view information so that decisions can be made starts with a vertical or horizontal view of such data elements.

Managing with KPIs includes setting targets (the desired level of performance) and tracking progress against that target. Managing with KPIs often means working to improve leading indicators that will later drive lagging benefits. Leading indicators are precursors of future success; lagging indicators show how successful the organization was at achieving results in the past.[33]

When curating, developing, or selecting KPIs, we do so with the expectation of extracting key data elements to not only review and make business decisions but to track and trend success. The following factors are key when determining metrics to track for business and financial management:

- Efficiency – Measurement of competencies
- Effectiveness – Measurement of workflow outcomes
- Quality – Measurement of the ability to meet predetermined standards
- Timeliness – Measurement of workflow and metric promptness
- Governance – Measurement of adherence to organizational rules
- Compliance – Identification of vulnerabilities and risk mitigation
- Behaviors – Identification of individual and organizational actions in comparison to expected standards
- Economics – Measurement of profit and loss trends
- Project Performance – Measurement of success in outlined project expectations
- Personnel Performance – Measurement of resource utilization and skill sets

Below are several business processes that are better managed by reviewing relevant metrics.

Business Process	Performance Metric	Description
Timeliness	Note Close Out Days	Average chart completion lag from DOS to Date of Submission
Economics	Time of Service Collections (TOS) %	Monies collected at the TOS as a % of owed balances
Quality	Readmission Rates	% of patients who are readmitted 30 days post-discharge

Exhibit 3.26 Selecting Metrics as Key Performance Indicators

With these factors in mind, we measure what we want to manage. Identifying and reviewing business processes that are vulnerable to internal or external factors is what drives the need for sharing results and findings with key stakeholders so that they may make informed decisions as well. Buffalo Medical Group (BMG), an MGMA Better Performer in Profitability and Value, was able to successfully improve measurements of KPIs by diversifying the manner in which results were shared with physicians. Information-sharing based on the preferred manner of the receiver is a priority in behavior changes.

Chief Financial Officer Deborah Bauer notes that BMG presents performance information to physicians in two ways: financially, via a dashboard, and clinically, via the practice's EHR. The former provides their monthly statements, their billing and collections information, and patient panel size for primary care providers. The latter allows providers to view their quality metrics goals, such as the Healthcare Effectiveness Data and Information Set (HEDIS), in value-based care programs such as MIPS. "We try to hone in and focus on the measures that matter," says Bauer, adding that HEDIS measures are quite important, because meeting them can bring in additional quality revenue outside fee schedules.[34]

Business processes will be positively or negatively impacted by the manner and timing in which we utilize the outcomes of selected metrics. Consistent process review will highlight vulnerabilities and opportunities within your organization. Formulating a process review strategy includes having an understanding of your organization's and workforce's current and future strengths and weaknesses. Without detailed reviews, obstacles and opportunities may look similar or will continue to be surface-level generalizations that cannot be resolved due to lack of actionable data.

As indicated in the above image, the accuracy of data is the initiation of transforming data into improvable business processes. The saying, "good data in, good data out," is relevant in this instance. The rate in which data/metrics are received drives the frequency of analysis. If data is extracted or available daily, then it can be measured daily. Some metrics do not need to be reviewed as frequently, so the rate in which it is analyzed might be monthly or quarterly. Workflows should

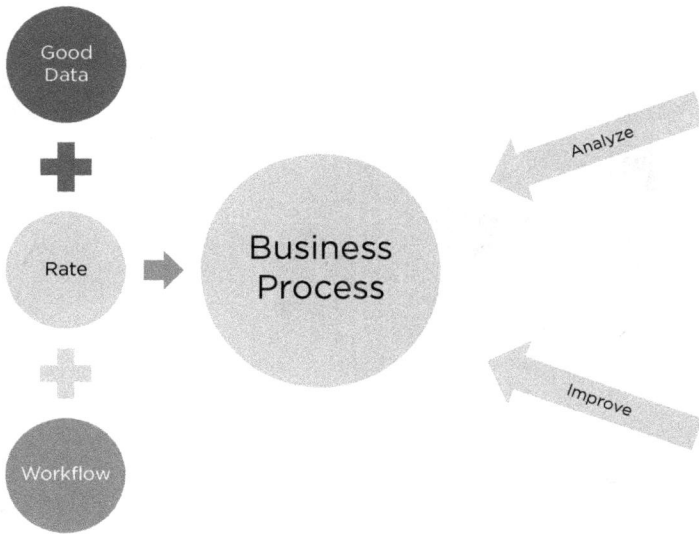

Exhibit 3.27 Business Process Improvement

align with business processes and standard operating procedures. Including metrics that allow for workflow review presents opportunities for improvement. Once business process KPIs have been selected, overall analysis may occur to validate required decisions based on factual data.

It would be unfathomable to have all of the wonderful information we've gathered from our KPIs and not take action or make decisions with that information. Failure to act is a disservice to the organization by ignoring red flags, process improvement or income opportunities as a result of information gathered from KPIs. To avoid data inertia, consider the outcomes of the data that has been analyzed. Factor in all risks. This would include risks that would result from inaction and risks as a result of errors identified. Formulate your plan based on evidence-based data which means identifying the outcomes, risk and workflows associated with each potential change.

How many of us have participated in the MGMA Compensation survey but never fully utilized the results? Obtaining decision-making data feeds an obligation to take action. Some decisions may require

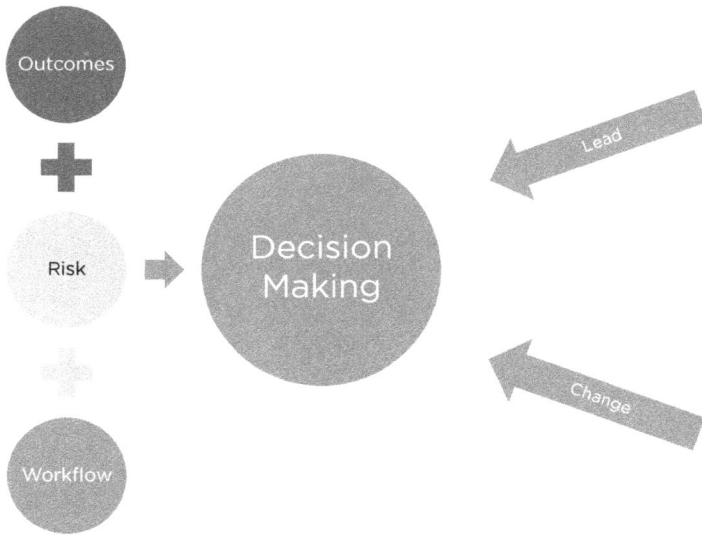

Exhibit 3.28 Decision Making Using KPIs

more information and planning than others. As an example, consider a medical practice that created a benchmark goal to have a 90% clean claims rate. This goal was established with the hopes that cashflow would increase and denials would decrease. In order to achieve this goal, the organization would need to have a 10% error rate. In this example, through data analysis, it was discovered that the clean claims rate (volume of claims accepted by payers without errors) was trending at 50%. This data informs us that the practice is not meeting its 90% clean claims expectation. Action taken to investigate the variance indicates that the claim scrubbing function for the clearinghouse was turned off due to cost. The decision to save on claims scrubbing costs resulted in a 40% drop in clean claims rate. The cost savings significantly lowered income. This is an opportunity to use data to take corrective action that will positively impact the practice's bottom line.

Prior to taking action, it's best to monitor a trend – but do not allow trends to become chronic problems, as they should be addressed as soon as the trend is identified. Evaluate the benefits of taking action. In this case, paying the claim scrubbing fees is more cost-effective than leaving it turned off. In the future, this type of decision could pass through an opportunity cost assessment prior to being operationalized.

Decisions that are made using KPI data include space renovations, equipment purchases to meet the demands of procedures/testing, satellite office expansion based on growth opportunities, increase or decrease in staffing based on performance, job complexity, and patient volumes. The data outcomes may point in the direction of relocation, outsourcing services, software/vendor changes, internal auditing or contract negotiations. KPIs fuel decision making by leveraging actionable data rather than projections or expectations. Stakeholders are much more open to decisions made on sound data than guesses.

Decisions that leverage KPIs may also be tracked back to an organizational business plan, recent or future regulatory changes, core competencies of your workforce, and provider workflow preferences.

Leaders rely on KPI data for strategic planning, business operations management, compliance and financial management. In leveraging KPIs for financial management we want to define our metrics, identify data that's available to us, select a timeframe for data capture, create a goal and benchmark results. Financial goals should be clear, concise and achievable. There will be industry best-practice benchmarks, but ultimately your organization will have unique financial motivations when selecting KPIs.

As seen in the below image, a healthcare organization may select payer-related KPIs to determine if payer participation is financially beneficial or whether it's necessary to negotiate fee schedule rates. Provider productivity KPIs shed light on predetermined compensation goals and determinations on equitable resource allocation.

Review the below KPIs to determine the financial decisions that could be extracted from this data.

Having KPIs in place is a key factor; however, benchmarking this data provides a full picture of data obtained. Benchmarking is the process of comparing and measuring areas of your organization with

Payer Mix & Payer Income
- Participation
- Fee Schedule Negotiation

Provider Productivity
- Compensation
- Resource distribution

Patient Age & Gender
- Preventive Services
- Track supply & equipment needs

Denial Reason Codes
- Appeal success rates
- Trending payer guidelines

Gross Charges
- Compared to Allowable amount
- Analysis of CDM

Unique Patient Visits
- Staffing needs
- Exam room utilization
- Appointment optimization

CPT Utilization
- Bell curve / coding accuracy
- Clinical Documentation Improvement

Diagnosis Utilization
- Engage high-risk patients
- Risk Adjustment

Referring Provider
- Patient sourcing
- Compliant Anti-Kickback marketing

Adjustments
- Collections performance
- Enhance specificity of adjustment codes

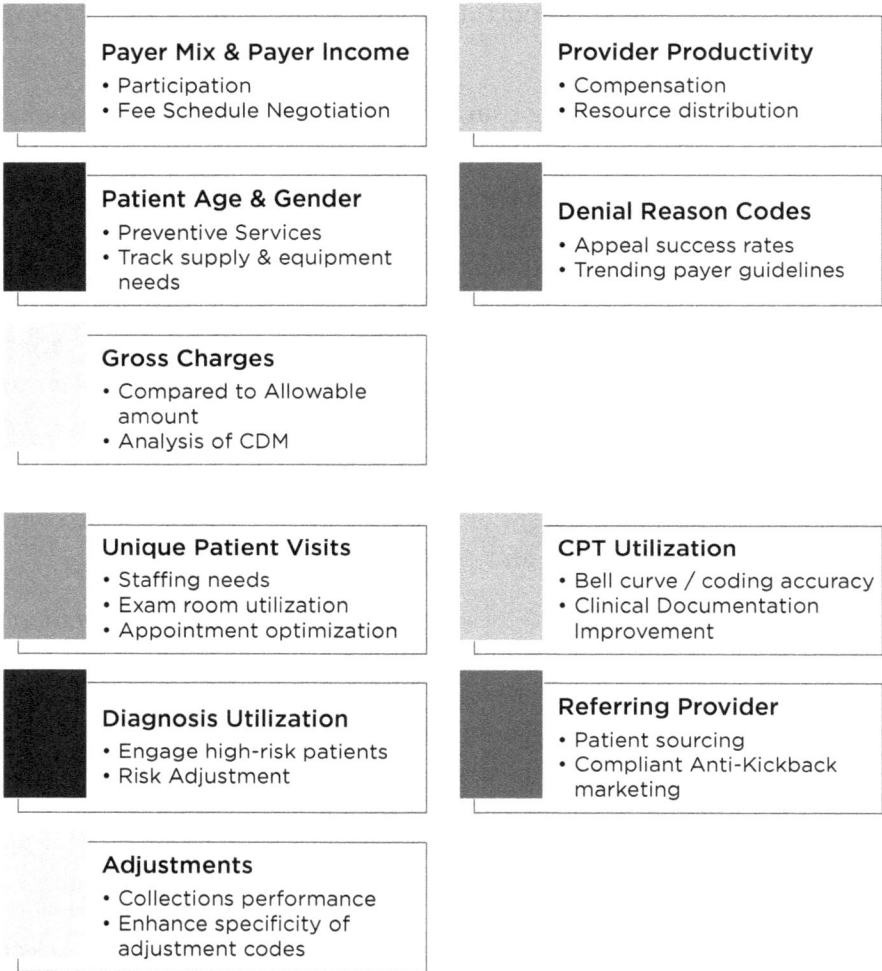

Exhibit 3.29 KPIs in Use for Financial Management

best practices. As we measure our success, we must also compare our results against a standard. In the above image, we can track adjustments – which are the contractual write-offs required when an organization accepts assignment. Adjustments could also be non-contractual write-offs due to inability to collect the full allowable amount. Both are metrics that should be tracked to monitor collections effectiveness and lost revenue. Utilizing industry best-practice benchmarks on both will inform a strength or weakness in this area.

When asked, "In what business areas did you utilize benchmarking data?" in an MGMA Stat poll, the most popular responses include compensation, staffing, finance (AR), patient access, and productivity.[35]

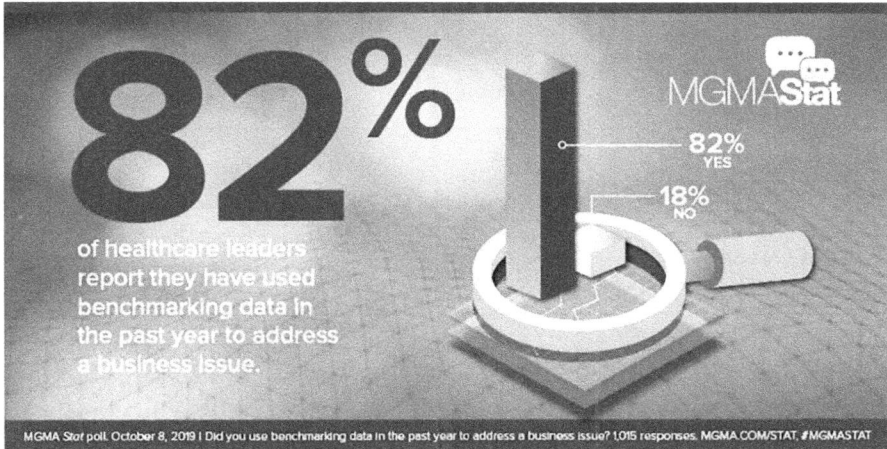

Exhibit 3.30 MGMA Stat Poll, Benchmarking Data Use

Benchmarking data is a vital component of optimizing financial management and developing achievable goals.

Beyond the Concept

Based on the below Profit and Loss Statement, answer the following questions:

1. What are current assets?   _____

2. What are current liabilities?   _____

3. What is current working capital?   _____

4. What is the monthly FFS revenues?   _____

5. What is the organization's largest liability? _____

We Fix You Medical Services
Profit and Loss Statement
June 1, 2022 – December 31, 2022

	Total
Revenue	
Fee-for-service Income	$1,875,444.00
Refunds	$1,255.00
Interest Earned	$250.00
Total Revenue	$1,876,949.00
Cost of Goods Sold	
Independent Contractors	$100,000.00
Expenses	
Rent	$85,000.00
Malpractice Insurance	$63,000.00
Liability, Cyber, and Workers Comp	$20,000.00
Medical Equipment	$45,000.00
Medical Supplies	$35,000.00
Software and Upgrades	$25,000.00
Office Supplies & Equipment	$20,000.00
Utilities, Telephone & Internet	$17,500.00
Dues, Licenses & Publications	$6,500.00
Professional Svcs: Attorney & Accountant	$7,000.00
Answering Service	$6,000.00
Payroll Expenses	
Payroll Processing	$4,200.00
Payroll Wages	$1,275,000.00
Payroll Taxes	$76,500.00
Total Operating Expenses	$1,785,700.00
Net Revenue	$91,249.00

Beyond the Concept Answers

1. $1,876,949.00
2. $1,785,700.00
3. $91,249.00
4. $312,574.00
5. Payroll

3.8 Case Study

For three consecutive months, an established multi-specialty group medical practice was having difficulty meeting monthly payroll. The physician partners were forced to accept partial paychecks to ensure all staff payroll obligations were met during the timeframe. During this time, there was a COVID-19 outbreak which required an all-hands-on-deck response due to an influx of patients requiring testing, vaccinations and virus symptoms. The partners became frustrated with the decrease in their take-home pay and they wanted answers about the inability to meet payroll.

During this time, several changes occurred:

(1) Members of the workforce became ill, leaving the organization severely short-staffed for physicians, nurses, medical assistants, billers and front office staff, creating burn-out as well as uncertainty on payout of sick-leave and other related benefits.

(2) The routine pre-visit check and pre-submission claim scrubbing functions were eliminated due to understaffing, causing claims to be denied.

(3) The organization's largest payer changed their reimbursement policies on COVID-19 vaccine administration and telehealth visit payments without the knowledge of the organization's remaining billing team.

(4) A vendor quoted bulk pricing discounts on PPE and other related supplies but did not honor the discount

due to an oversight in contract interpretation, which left the organization liable for higher than anticipated supply expenses.

Working capital management requires routine oversight of assets and liabilities. The solutions used to bring the organization back to a stance of financial stability included making contact with the state and federal Department of Labor to obtain guidance on how to approach short-term disability and sick-pay during the public health emergency. This guidance allowed the organization to create an internal policy that was then followed whenever members of the workforce needed to be out of the office due to personal or family sickness. The policy assisted the organization with managing payroll expenses.

Although the organization had the technology to automate the pre-visit and pre-claim submission processes, staff push-back had prevented going live with these functions in the past. Leadership researched the already included features, obtained training for all required staff, tested several claims and immediately went live with automating processes that reduced related denials by 45%.

Contact was made with the payer whose reimbursement guidelines had been changed. The organization obtained a written copy of the new policy, corrected impacted claims and resubmitted them. Claims edits were created internally to scrub claims against the payer's guidelines prior to passing through the clearinghouse. As a result, 85% of resubmitted claims were paid and future claims were paid without challenge.

The practice manager was able to renegotiate the vendor's supply agreement to reduce rates to the original agreed-upon amount. A supply inventory control process was implemented, notifying leadership when supplies were at 40% to initiate the reorder process.

Notes

1. https://nahri.org/membership/ethics
2. https://www.fiercehealthcare.com/finance/funding-down-56-healthcare-ai-stand-apart-market-volatility

3. https://www.hfma.org/topics/hfm/2020/may/8-hallmarks-of-a-successful -healthcare-venture-capital-program.html

4. False Claims Act, 31 U.S.C. § 3729 – 3733 (1863).

5. Anti Kickback Statute, 42 U.S.C. § 1320a-7b (1972).

6. Physician Self-Referral, 42 U.S.C. § 1395nn (1989).

7. Civil Monetary Penalties, 42 U.S.C. § 1320a-7a

8. Civil Monetary Penalties, 42 U.S.C. § 1320a-7a (2010).

9. Occupational Safety and Health Standards, 29 U.S.C. § 1910 (1974).

10. https://www.cdc.gov/chronicdisease/about/foa/1815/index.htm

11. https://www.cdc.gov/chronicdisease/about/foa/1815/index.htm

12. https://EMMA.maryland.gov

13. https://www.commbuys.com/bso/

14. www.greenbookdc.com

15. 42 CFR Part 411 [CMS-1720-F] RIN 0938-AT64 (Pages 40-41). https://public -inspection.federalregister.gov/2020-26140.pdf

16. 42 CFR Part 411 [CMS-1720-F] RIN 0938-AT64 (Page 194). https://public inspection.federalregister.gov/2020-26140.pdf

17. https://www.modernhealthcare.com/article/20120106/BLOGS01/301069983/a -closer-look-at-hospital-write-offs

18. https://www.beckershospitalreview.com/finance/margins-remain-narrow-for -us-hospitals.html

19. https://www.aha.org/fact-sheets/2020-01-06-fact-sheet-uncompensated-hospital -care-cost

20. https://www.mhaonline.com/blog/service-line-structures-in-healthcare

21. https://oamp.od.nih.gov/division-of-financial-advisory-services/indirect-cost -branch/indirect-cost-submission/indirect-cost-definition-and-example

22. https://www.healthcatalyst.com/insights/healthcare-activity-based-costing -transforming-cost

23. https://www.healthcatalyst.com/success_stories/risk-based-contracting-partners -healthcare

24. https://www.cms.gov/newsroom/fact-sheets/calendar-year-cy-2022-medicare -physician-fee-schedule-final-rule?mkt_tok=MTQ0LUFNSi02MzkAAAGAg W0BtWi2I7XajN6WVG8JyLyMjRrwNrNlZssDEtBHHbCzUJgeRuNO_zo SFryuxwRnaXQDvuDlL-yrBSljAQbI38XAD_8jLHiXJ-MACTgo

25. https://www.whitehouse.gov/wp-content/uploads/2023/01/SAP-H.R.-382-H.J. -Res.-7.pdf.

26. https://data.cdc.gov/NCHS/Telemedicine-Use-in-the-Last-4-Weeks/h7xa-837u

27. https://www.cms.gov/files/zip/list-telehealth-services-calendar-year-2023-updated-11022022.zip

28. https://www.novitas-solutions.com/webcenter/portal/MedicareJL/FeeLookup

29. 16 Potential Key Performance Indicators. Beckers. https://www.beckershospital review.com/strategic-planning/16-potential-key-performance-indicators-for-hospitals.html#:~:text=Key%20performance%20indicators%20are%20defined,processes%20and%20reflect%20strategic%20performance.

30. https://www.h4-technology.com/our-solution/claims-data-management/payer-mix/

31. https://www.mgma.com/data/data-stories/the-kpis-that-matter-most-in-medical-practices-co

32. https://www.forbes.com/sites/forbesbusinesscouncil/2021/07/26/the-value-of-key-performance-indicators/?sh=14376ef64231

33. https://kpi.org/KPI-Basics

34. https://www.mgma.com/practice-resources/health-information-technology/mgma-better-performers-buffalo-medical-group-embra

35. MGMA Stat poll. October 8, 2019. https://www.mgma.com/data/data-stories/benchmarking-for-success

Chapter 4

Compliance Efforts

Managing compliance in the revenue cycle means more than knowing existing rules. It also requires you to stay updated on the impact of new and pending legislation. The challenge with educating to compliance is that the rules have often changed by the time the paper's been printed on. In this section, our goal is to teach you how to recognize when new regulations are coming, how to identify where components therein may impact your revenue cycle, and what your options are in those situations. If you've been implementing changes for the No Surprises Act, then you know the impact legislation can have on a healthcare entity. Keeping abreast of changes makes a significant difference in how your facility is able to respond when they go into effect.

As with any compliance effort, always make sure to verify the current requirements with the appropriate governing bodies. Consult legal counsel without delay whenever you have questions about regulatory guidance and adherence to pending legislation.

Let's walk through a few pieces of legislation impacting the industry now, discuss how to maintain tax exempt status and consider the impact of legislation on finance.

4.1 Historical Legislation with Financial Impacts

History is flush with examples of legislative acts absolutely rocking the healthcare industry. For example, 1935 saw the introduction of the Social Security Act, which continues to serve as a significant foundation for maternal and child health. In 1965, Medicaid and Medicare were added under the umbrella of the Social Security Act. Together, these programs constitute a significant portion of the payer mix for most organizations. Fast forward to 1996. HIPAA created a significant amount of administrative burden, but it also promoted the portability and protection of personal health information. Fourteen years later, the Affordable Care Act (ACA) was passed. The cumulative impact of these landmark laws is the expansion of health coverage and more patient ownership of personal data.

Reflecting on these pieces of legislation and their decades-long impact should cement the importance of tracking legislation as a regular task. Here is what we need to know to anticipate and prepare for prospective changes.

Annual Compliance Tips

Reviewing rules prior to finalization is a fantastic way to anticipate what may be coming. Knowing the process, even at a high level, can impact your ability to prepare.

Important Distinctions

- **Proposed Rules** are issued by CMS and other federal/state bodies to let you know what they are planning to do in the upcoming term. Every year CMS issues a host of proposed rules impacting providers, hospitals, and administrative staff across the industry.
- **Comment Periods** give interested parties 60 days to respond to proposed rules before CMS evaluates the responses and makes a final decision.
- **Final Rules** do not have further comments to that rule considered.

As mentioned above, there is first the release of the proposed rule (PR), followed by a comment period, CMS review, and then the release of the final rule (FR), which contains responses to comments submitted. All of the PRs and FRs can be located online free of charge at the Federal Register.[1] To see what this looks like for a given rule, let's consider the annually released CMS Physician Fee Schedule (PFS). The timing depicted below is pretty typical.

Exhibit 4.1 CMS Rules Process

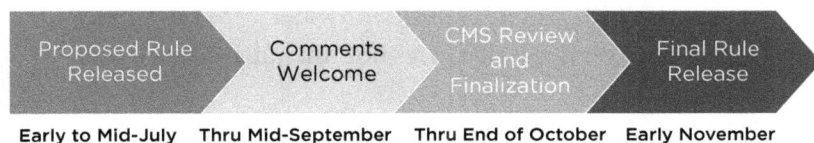

Proposed Rule Released	Comments Welcome	CMS Review and Finalization	Final Rule Release
Early to Mid-July	Thru Mid-September	Thru End of October	Early November

These dates vary when challenges arise, sometimes falling earlier or later than these windows, but this gives an indication of when you should be looking for proposed or finalized changes for the upcoming year.

Operationalizing Regulations

Once you've evaluated upcoming changes, you can take action. For example, look at changes that came into effect in 2022 and the methods used to optimize operations in response to these changes.

Exhibit 4.2 Rule changes and actions

Rule Change	Action
Stark Law: Relaxations allow greater collaboration between entities	Evaluate collaborative opportunities for value-based program participation.
Information Blocking Rule: Creates penalties for delays in providing access to patient PHI	Assess records release processes and the method of receiving records requests. Optimize protocols before this goes into effect.
Anti-Kickback Statute: New and updated safe harbors put into place	Evaluate opportunities to allow IT expense payments or outsource care coordination staff.

Though this is a short list of changes to regulations, it illustrates the opportunities. When you have changes to regulations, there will generally be new restrictions, but you should also look for the opportunities that new regulations may provide.

4.2 Tackling Price Transparency and Surprise Billing

To provide a more recent example of impactful legislation, let's take a quick dive into the No Surprises Act (NSA) of 2021. The NSA went into effect January 1, 2022, and included three primary components: billing regulations, price transparency, and patient billing protections.

- Billing Regulations: This section regulates the definition of a surprise bill, which facilities/provider types it applies to, and any services that are not included under this mandate.
- Price Transparency: This component defines the provider's responsibility to provide cost information to the patient in advance, including alternative options available.
- Patient Protections: Notably, if surprise medical bills (as defined by HHS) are issued to patients, the patient will be held harmless, and the facility may be at risk for violating the NSA.

Among others, this regulation includes regulations on:

- Applicable providers
- Dispute resolution processes (patient and payer)
- The provision of estimates in good faith to patients

The largest financial impacts of this rule come down to three things:

1. The prohibition of balance-billing patients for services rendered by out-of-network providers at in-network facilities
2. The requirement to negotiate directly with payers for total reimbursement of out-of-network services or go through the federal independent dispute resolution (IDR) arbitration process
3. The administrative burden associated with providing accurate Good Faith Estimates (GFEs) and all related tasks

Balance Billing Exception

There are certain circumstances in which the patient can be balance billed under the NSA. To meet these requirements, non-ancillary OON providers at in-network facilities must:

1. Notify the patient that the care is out-of-network

2. Offer the patient other in-network options at that facility

3. Provide an estimated cost of care to the patient

4. Receive the patient's confirmation that they elect to continue with the OON provider

If all of the above steps have been met, the provider can balance bill the patient without risk of violating the NSA.

The IDR Timeline

If a provider cannot balance a bill and feels the out-of-network payment rate from the payer is unacceptable, the provider does have the option to initiate a federal IDR process arbitrated by federally certified arbiters. It is a long process and it comes with associated fees per determination. The timeline from start to finish can be anywhere from 60-120 days after the notice of payment or denial from the payer. An example of how far the timeline can potentially reach is reflected below:

Exhibit 4.3 IDR Timeline

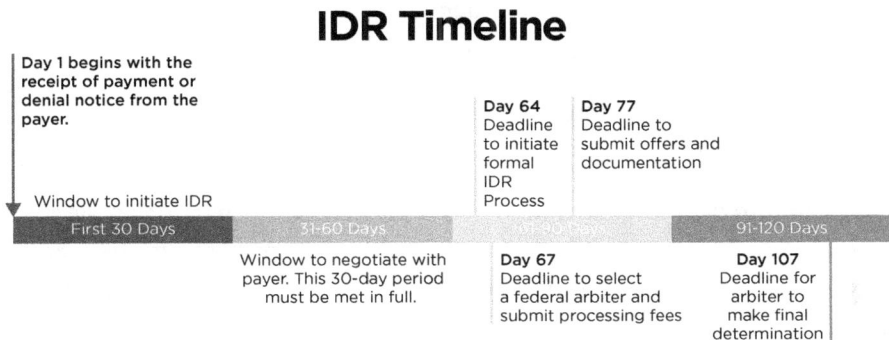

IDR Timeline

Day 1 begins with the receipt of payment or denial notice from the payer.

Window to initiate IDR

Day 64 Deadline to initiate formal IDR Process

Day 77 Deadline to submit offers and documentation

First 30 Days | 31-60 Days | 61-90 Days | 91-120 Days

Window to negotiate with payer. This 30-day period must be met in full.

Day 67 Deadline to select a federal arbiter and submit processing fees

Day 107 Deadline for arbiter to make final determination

Keep in mind that the No Surprises Act is but one piece of legislation that impacts the healthcare industry. Therefore, it is imperative that leaders who aspire to achieve success and long-term financial stability remain attentive to regulatory changes.

4.3 Maintaining Tax-Exempt Status

No healthcare organization wants the IRS challenging its tax-exempt status. The defense is a solid offense that includes understanding and adhering to IRS guidelines along with regular monitoring of transactions for risk management. In this complicated area of tax law, healthcare organizations would do well to have advice from tax professionals knowledgeable in state and federal laws related to tax-exempt status, which often involves the regulation of tax-exempt medical items such as supplies and diagnostic equipment. Although it's important to follow IRS guidelines, also check with your state to see if there are overlapping or contradicting exemptions. Note: just by the nature of their services, healthcare organizations are often, and sometimes erroneously, believed to be tax-exempt.

The typical IRS tax-exempt recognition is outlined in Section 501 (c)(3). The IRS has an effective Operational Test to assist you in ensuring your organization meets the requirements of Section 501(c)(3):[2]

1. Requirement to operate exclusively for tax-exempt purposes
2. Prohibition against inurement
3. Prohibition against becoming an action organization
4. Prohibition against substantial private benefit

The second factor in the operational test is inurement. "IRC 501(c)(3) expressly provides that to qualify for exemption, no part of an organization's net earnings shall inure in whole or in part to the benefit of private shareholders or individuals. Private shareholders or individuals are defined as persons having a personal and private interest in the activities of the organization."[3] Healthcare organizations that regularly conduct internal inurement audits will be able to mitigate the risk of non-compliance with tax-exempt requirements. As part of an inurement review, it is essential to outline physician-owner compensation packages and methods used for determination, as well as to conduct a review to determine if excessive private benefit is occurring.

Some of the key tax-exempt indicators are: Community Benefit, Charitable and Uncompensated Care. The value of charitable services provided annually as a percentage of gross income is factored into tax-exempt status, which is why it's critical to track these numbers through adjustment/write-off codes for end-of-year reporting. Although state Medicaid beneficiaries are covered for approved services, we want to track the percentage that Medicaid represents in our adjustments and revenue to monitor the amount of potentially indigent patients who may have Social Determinants of Health (SDoH) requiring additional uncompensated supportive services.

Exhibit 4.4 Charity Care Adjustment Report

Charity Care Adjustment Report January 1, 2022 – December 31, 2022		
Adjustment Code	Description	Amount
MCD	State Medicaid Contractual	$550,000.00
UNINS	Uninsured	$75,000.00
FINHARD	Financial Hardship	$55,000.00
SFS	Sliding Fee Scale	$35,000.00
Total		$165,000.00

When managing uncompensated care revenues or losses, the importance of having published policies is essential. Patients, family members and staff need to be aware of the organization's participation with Medicare and Medicaid as well as sliding fee scale arrangements for eligible individuals. The eligibility criteria for a sliding fee scale must be in writing and explained to those who may qualify. A financial policy should also describe the availability of these types of financial arrangements as well as a fair debt collection practice.

According to the IRS, maintaining status as a non-profit can be just as easy as losing it.[4]

The basic components of maintaining tax-exempt status are:

1. Activities should be directed toward exempt purposes, i.e., not for private benefit.

2. Lobbying activities, though permitted, should not be a substantial portion of efforts.

3. Participating in political campaigning is strictly prohibited.

4. Unrelated business income (UBI) should be carefully monitored. There are certain exemptions as to what counts against a non-profit. Carefully discuss these areas with your accountant.

5. Complete annual reports on time.

6. Perform the exempt activities that are dictated in the IRS application that you submitted when initially seeking exempt status.

For more information on maintaining tax-exempt status, the IRS provides additional resources:

- Tax information for charities & other non-profits and the IRS' free exempt organization newsletter, the EO Update, may be found at https://www.irs.gov/
- Phone forum presentations on tax-exempt issues may be found at https://www.stayexempt.irs.gov/

Losing tax-exempt status can be devastating to an organization. If you have a tax-exempt status, make sure to perform regular reviews with your CPA and legal counsel. Establish a non-profit board that can develop the overall strategy, drive adherence, and monitor potential areas of concern.

Each state has statutes of limitations on these types of audits. The audit timeframe may increase in circumstances in which non-compliance is detected and requires investigation on issues like significant over- or underpayments, inaccurate tax return data and fraudulent activities. Documentation is critical. Make sure to document all donations received, all activities performed, any unrelated business income, lobbying efforts, etc. Keep in mind that unrelated business income is subject to tax, so that must be documented separately and clearly for your accountant to properly file. If you fall into non-compliance with your tax-exempt status, you can lose your status or have a heavy fine levied by the IRS.

An organization created by a physician to operate a medical clinic may apply for exemption under IRC 501(c)(3). Under Rev. Proc. 90-27, 1990-1 C.B. 514, Section 5, Standards for Issuing Rulings or Determination Letters with Respect to Exempt Status, we would need detailed information as part of the application to provide assurances concerning the absence of private benefit and inurement.

Questions to elicit this information would include:

- Is there a community board of directors? If not, how will the organization make decisions to ensure the clinic is operating for a public rather than a private purpose? For example, are patient services available to the community or only to the physician's private practice patients?
- What is the physician's compensation package? How was it determined? Were comparable data applicable to similarly situated physicians utilized?
- If the organization leases, purchases, or shares facilities, employees, equipment, or its name with the physician's own medical practice, what are the terms of any such arrangement? How does the organization ensure that these arrangements do not result in excessive private benefit?

Beyond the Concept

In a medical office or facility, your approach and dedication to compliance efforts will directly impact your success and longevity. Creating a compliance checklist and working through that checklist is the best way to ensure organizational compliance, but then what? True mastery of healthcare compliance means continuous improvement; it means you didn't stop at the end of the checklist and say "that's done." Instead, you thought "what's next," or "what else can we do?" New pieces of regulatory guidance and legislation are published annually by a variety of oversight agencies. Engaging in government affairs and advocacy efforts will help you stay ahead of prospective changes that can impact your facility.

Regularly reviewing healthcare news, policy updates, and proposed legislation can seem like a daunting task, but there are a few easy ways to build this into your routine:

1. Subscribe and listen to industry-related podcasts
2. Bookmark relevant industry news websites and scan the headlines daily, digging in where relevant
3. Read the news summaries provided by industry and specialty associations
4. Participate in government affairs committees

By keeping your finger on the pulse of the industry, you will begin to think in predictive ways that will benefit your future efforts. We are only capable of working with our current level of knowledge. You can either do a great service to yourself and your organization by increasing your knowledge in these areas, or you can do a great disservice.

4.5 Case Study

In 2013, Astellas Pharma US Inc. and Amgen, Inc. developed what has been seen both before and since at many healthcare facilities: a copay waiver/assistance program. Though the intent here appears noble, waiving copays and deductibles can be seen as a type of bribe or coercive tactic to prevent your patients from going elsewhere. This in turn can result in hefty fines and enforcement actions from the Office of the Inspector General (OIG) and/or the Department of Justice (DOJ).

This is what happened to Astellas and Amgen. We often see facilities waiving copays because they don't know the consequences. Astellas and Amgen allegedly went one step further by working with copay foundations to create a steady stream of copay funds for patients who were consumers of their own medications.

Astellas and Amgen's position was that they offered donations to copay foundations to specifically support patients who needed these high-cost medications which treated conditions such as hyperthyroidism and prostate cancer.

The DOJ's position was that "the companies' payments to the foundations were not 'donations,' but rather were kickbacks. According to United States Attorney General, Andrew E. Lelling, these kickbacks "undermined the structure of the Medicare program and illegally subsidized the high costs of the companies' drugs at the expense of American taxpayers. We will keep pursuing these cases until pharmaceutical companies stop engaging in this kind of behavior."[5]

The full details of the allegations made against Astellas and Amgen are available elsewhere. The primary takeaway here is that after nearly six years of evaluation and consideration, in 2019 the two companies settled for over $124 million, or the equivalent of almost 2.5 million $50 copays. Each company also entered a five-year compliance integrity agreement with the OIG which requires that they implement measures, controls and monitoring designed to promote independence from any patient assistance program to which they donate.

Notes

1. https://www.federalregister.gov

2. https://www.irs.gov/charities-non-profits/charitable-hospitals-general-requirements-for-tax-exemption-under-section-501c3

3. Gitterman JE and Friedlander M. https://www.irs.gov/pub/irs-tege/eotopicc04.pdf

4. How to lose your 501(c)(3) tax-exempt status (without really trying). https://www.irs.gov/pub/irs-tege/How%20to%20Lose%20Your%20Tax%20Exempt%20Status.pdf

5. United States Department of Justice. https://www.justice.gov/opa/pr/two-pharmaceutical-companies-agree-pay-total-nearly-125-million-resolve-allegations-they-paid. Accessed 1.16.23.

Chapter 5

Patient Outreach

The successful financial oversight of a healthcare organization would be incomplete without inclusion of the patient within the process. Yes, we need to collect patient balances, but we also need our patient population to be educated about the financial aspects of their care. Patients who lack this understanding will also lack the motivation to prioritize payment of medical bills or, worse, avoid medical treatment altogether. The concept of patient outreach is self-explanatory but often overlooked. Our best approach to patient outreach is to meet patients where they are. Are patients visiting your website? Meet them there. Are patients logging into the patient portal? Meet them there. Are patients on social media? Again, meet them there. There is an entire science behind reinventing payment options, approaching the design of patient statements and prediction collections. All of these areas are critical for improving the collection of patient payments, increasing patient engagement and decreasing attrition due to bad debt.

5.1 Reinventing Payment Options

It is in your practice's best interest to have standard, documented guidelines that dictate company policy on patient copays, payment arrangements, financial hardship qualifications, and patient balances both in and out of collections.

<u>Best Practices Include:</u>

- Send clear patient statements
- Abide by FDCPA if required
- Educate staff on collections
- Understand opportunities to collect
- Maintain HIPAA compliance
- Remove payment obstacles
- Automate payment options

The Federal Debt Collections Practices Act (FDCPA) only applies directly to "debt collectors," and any creditor who is attempting to collect debts for itself and under its own name is not considered a "debt collector." Nonetheless, any employees responsible for collecting debt on behalf of the practice should be educated on FDCPA, as these standards provide a good basis for collections decision-making.

Many employees do not feel comfortable collecting past-due balances from patients. The key in these situations is to thoroughly train and educate your staff in "how" and "why." By educating the front desk and any reception staff on the importance of collections and the role they play in the overall revenue cycle, you will empower them to act effectively on behalf of the practice while maintaining good relationships with the patients.

For face-to-face collections, make sure staff is aware of how to implement appropriate HIPAA privacy considerations. If the lobby is too small to provide privacy, meet with patients in an empty exam room or quiet office to discuss their balances.

During the conversation, remove the provider from the discussion. It is ideal if you can offer multiple payment options, explain balances, and obtain a commitment for payment. It is also very important not to appear confrontational, as many patients will find this topic emotional. Conversations can be improved by stating facts, staying objective, and leaving the patient with something in writing that outlines their financial obligations to the organization.

When attempting to collect from a patient, it is very helpful to have as many methods of payment available as possible. At a minimum, the practice should accept cash, money orders, and credit cards. As there is a generation of individuals who still prefer to write checks, consider accepting those as well. It is also convenient if you can offer payment processing through the patient portal. Make sure staff have information on the nearest ATM handy. The practice can also offer automated payment deductions for large balances. If several methods of payment are available to the patient, you remove excuses from the patient, thereby increasing your chances of collection.

Time of Service Collections

When the patient is present in the office or on the phone, there is a greater ability to collect their financial responsibilities. Best practice reminders for TOS collections include:

- Optimizing every patient interaction to collect outstanding payments
- Encouraging collaboration between the front desk and billing department
- Educating staff on collecting past-due balances
- Monitoring staff collection and evaluating performance
- Creating processes that drive staff accountability for past due balance collections

The Psychology of Patient Statements

There is a method to the design and submission of patient statements that can increase the likelihood of collection. Best practices include:

1. Including pertinent information with clear messaging. Minimize the use of procedural codes and complex code descriptions
2. Setting a threshold for amounts that are less than the cost of sending statements
3. Making a minimum of three attempts to collect

4. Sending patient statements as quickly as possible after the claim has been adjudicated

5. Sending statements the way patients want to receive them and allowing them to opt-in to paper or electronic statements

6. Consolidating the most important components quickly: Amount Due, Due Date, Payment Methods

Exhibit 5.1 Examples of successful patient statements

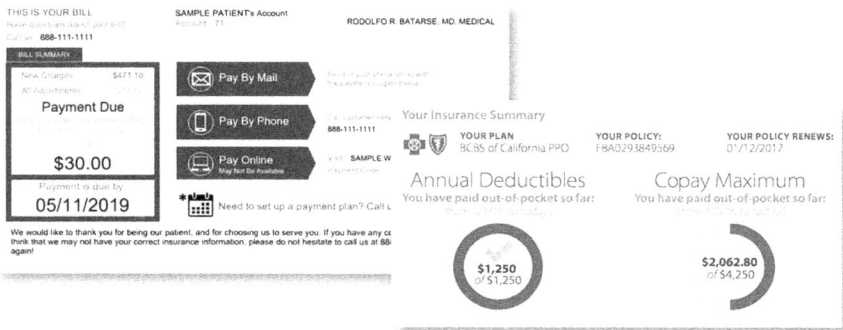

The above examples are from Mail My Statements, a billing and payment solutions company.[1] They reflect visually appealing patient statements. What you can see here is that the patient has an easy method for identifying payment amounts, deductibles, copay maximums, and payment methods. The easier you make it for patients to comply, the more likely they will.

HFMA's Patient-Friendly Billing

Healthcare Financial Management Association (HFMA) created the "Patient Friendly Billing Project"[2] after conducting extensive research and focus groups among patients and healthcare providers. The consensus was clear: patient billing is a significant problem for patients and providers. Consumers want a healthcare financial communications process that is clear, concise, correct, and patient-friendly. HFMA's Patient Friendly Billing Project defines its goals as follows:

- **Clear**: All financial communications should be easy to understand and written in clear language. Patients should be able to quickly determine what they need to do with the communication.
- **Concise**: The bills should contain just the right amount of detail necessary to communicate the message.
- **Correct**: The bills or statements should not include estimates of liabilities, incomplete information, or errors.
- **Patient-Friendly:** The needs of patients and family members should be paramount when designing administrative processes and communications.

General Improvement Practices

1. **Automate collection where possible.** This means obtaining consent from the patient to charge their card or bank account monthly with a certain amount. Be very clear with patients where they will be charged and how much will be charged. Do not add items to the patient's payment plan without their consent.

2. **Communicate regularly.** Send invoices to patients monthly. Increase the urgency in the formatting and layout as days in A/R increase. Notify clearly before sending to collections. When patients are set up on payment plans, send monthly reminders, especially if their payment will be automatically deducted.

3. **Set standards.** Don't allow unreasonable plans. If a patient has a balance of $1,500, paying $5/month is not reasonable.

4. **Collect something at setup.** To set up payment plans and show the intention to collect, it's important to collect the first payment at the time of payment plan setup. This affirms to the patient that the practice is serious about collection, and to the practice that the patient intends to pay.

5. **Offer multiple methods of payment.** Do you accept cash, credit cards, bank drafts? The more options patients have the more likely they are to make their payments.

5.2 Predictive Patient Collections

A frequent misunderstanding across the industry is that we don't know the amounts due from patients ahead of time. This misunderstanding typically stems from the generally complex nature of the healthcare industry and payer contract language which varies greatly by payer and plan.

There are a variety of resources to help support predictive patient collections: software tools, embedded predictive analytics tools, etc. In the absence of these tools, you can still have and implement predictive patient collection strategies. As with so many of the critical financial processes, success here begins with the front desk – more specifically, at the point of appointment scheduling. This is the interaction with the patient where we gather their insurance payer and plan information. This portion of the patient's demographic information is where we can gather insight on prospective patient expenses.

Getting Started with Predictive Patient Collections

Options for identifying patient responsibilities:

1. Electronic
   a. Embedded Benefit Management Tool in PM/EHR
   b. Third-Party Benefit Verification Tool to login to
   c. Algorithmic Estimations based on Historical Payer Payment Data from ERAs
2. Manual
   a. Manual Payer Portal Search
   b. Calling Payer Directly
   c. Reviewing Patient's Card Details
   d. Reviewing Payer Plan Details Online

Standard Policies to Consider

1. Copays – Always collect up front at check-in. An attempt to collect copays must be made at least three times to remain

in compliance with CMS and other payers. The patient has a greater sense of urgency to pay their copay when they are right in front of you and the effort/cost to collect is much less than invoicing for the copayment collection.

2. Procedures – Always perform a financial review for high-cost services and procedures. This is required for out-of-network services with the No Surprises Act, but it's also a collections best practice. Prior to scheduling procedures/surgeries, review the patient's benefits and anticipated out-of-pocket expenses for the procedure and collect the payment in advance. This will help improve collections efforts, inform the patient of their cost responsibilities, reduce procedure no shows, and reduce the likelihood of writing off entire procedures as bad debt down the road.

3. Deductibles – Have a plan for patients with high deductibles. This means creating realistic payment policies and options that are given to patients in advance of the services being rendered so they can determine if the cost is worth it or if they need financial support. Have a plan for the financial support as well.

   These policies will help to standardize your internal processes while informing the patient community that your facility will give them critical financial information in advance but that you also expect payment for services rendered.

In the days of paper charts, we performed chart prep several days before the patient's appointment, and could document anticipated patient expenses for collection by the front desk at that time. Usually, the billing department reviewed the patient's record and benefits and documented the amount to collect in red and highlighted it on the visit superbill before paperclipping it to the patient chart. We gained a lot moving away from paper charts, but we lost some things too. We need to get back to the "chart prep" process. Maybe it needs a new name, but the goal is the same. We need to make sure everything the provider needs is in there and in order, and we need to make sure we've communicated everything we need to the front desk so they can obtain it during check-in.

Complications

Unfortunately, the above processes, like everything else in this industry, has complications that create exceptions to the rule. For example, in 2022 several payers began documenting in their provider agreements that collecting payments in advance of claim adjudication would constitute a breach of contract, a practice that effectively prohibited the collection of any copays or high-cost procedure balances for a few weeks after the patient was seen. The challenge in this situation is that the patient then lacks the urgency to pay. For patients with high deductibles, if they choose to no longer respond to requests for payment, the facility may spend months or years attempting to collect, along with the expenses of that effort.

If you read through chapter three, you understand not only the importance of compliance, but also the importance of advocacy. For these reasons it is a strategic necessity to thoroughly read and understand your payer contracts prior to implementing the predictive patient collection policies listed above.

Beyond the Concept

Achieving long-term financial stability requires patient engagement, and the best way to engage patients is to make complex financial processes easy to understand. If it is challenging for patients to identify how to make payments, why payments are due, and how to navigate online payment portals, they disengage from the process. Understanding this as a concept is easy, but genuinely moving beyond it means taking the time to look at every process in your organization from the patient's perspective. Regularly assess your patient-facing financial processes from the patient's perspective to identify improvement opportunities. The following assessment may be performed internally and/or given to patients for input. As you begin to assess interaction points as opportunities for improvement through the lens of the patient, you are beginning to move beyond the concept.

Exhibit 5.2 Patient Engagement and Access Assessment

Patient-Facing Process	Self-Rating 1-5 1 needs Improvement, 5 Exceeds Expectations	Total Score	Improvement Opportunities
Patient Portal access and registration			
Patient Portal navigation			
Accessibility to online Financial Policy			
Online payment options			
Online accessibility support options for the hearing-impaired			
Wait time to speak with staff regarding invoices			
Staff ability to collect patient balances during in-person and telephone interactions			
Accessibility of online medical records in accordance with CURES Act			
Online guidance regarding No Surprises Act & Good Faith Estimates			

5.4 Case Study

This case study is a bit different as it's being recounted from the patient's perspective. A patient in the Midwest with an eye-related injury reached out to a local ophthalmology practice for assistance. We will call this patient Alishia to maintain confidentiality. On the scheduling call, Alishia was informed that she can be seen within the hour, but since she hasn't yet met her deductible, she will need to pay for the visit in full. The employee, who we will refer to as Melanie, relayed over the phone that the contracted rate for her insurance was $270 for new patient visits, and that amount would need to be paid at check-in.

At this point, the patient has a high level of urgency, she cannot see out of one eye and doesn't want to go to the emergency room, which entails a longer wait and higher expense. She agrees to the expense, schedules the visit and goes into the office. At check-in she offers to pay the amount she was given over the phone and is told the amount will be collected after her appointment. Alishia is seen promptly, treated quickly, and prescribed medication for immediate relief. At this point, her perception of this facility is very positive. It seems to be a well-oiled machine. The provider walks her to the check-out desk. This impresses her, as she recalls usually having to navigate there on her own at the completion of a visit.

She stops at the check-out desk expecting to submit payment but is again prevented from doing so. The check-out staff informs her that they don't take payments at check-out. She recounts her discussion with Melanie to the check-out staff, but she can't recall Melanie's name. The staff call in the front desk supervisor who says, "Ma'am, if you owe anything we will bill you. You can go." With quite a bit of confusion, she again relays her conversation with Melanie. At this point the staff is exhibiting obvious frustration and sternly tells Alishia that they will bill her for the visit.

Approximately 90 days later, Alishia received the invoice in the mail post-adjudication. Unsurprisingly, she owed $270 since she hadn't yet met her deductible. She went online to the website to submit payment to the office but could not pay online without setting up a patient portal account. She clicked to confirm her desire to submit for an account and completed two screens of registration data before she was asked for a registration code. Clicking on the information icon informed her, after almost 15 minutes trying to pay her bill, that she could only get this code in person at the office.

This entire situation could have been avoided if collection had been permitted in *any way* while the patient was in the office. The most infuriating part from the patient's perspective is that someone in the office was absolutely right about what she owed. After speaking with the office manager, it was identified that "Melanie is new and shouldn't have been giving out that information," for which the manager apologized. This fermented the patient's frustration with this facility. She resolved to never return to the office.

There are so many hurdles to successful financial engagement in this situation. Key takeaways:

- An excellent clinical experience does not supersede a frustrating payment experience
- An uninformed staff is a detriment to the revenue cycle
- Informed patients are more likely to make attempts to pay their bills
- The harder the payment process is, the more frustrating it is for the patient, and the less likely it is that they will submit payments

Notes

1. Mail My Statements blog. https://mailmystatements.com/2019/06/05/the-psychology -behind-a-visually-appealing-patient-statement/. Accessed on 1.16.23.

2. Patient Friendly Billing® is a proprietary trademark of Healthcare Financial Management Association, copyright© 2019, Healthcare Financial Management Association, all rights reserved.

Chapter 6

Revenue Cycle Integrity:
Bringing It All Together

The integrity of your revenue cycle isn't composed solely of accurate demographic entries or clean claims submission rates. Revenue Cycle Integrity (RCI) looks at your entire revenue cycle: past, present, and potential future. RCI uses this to establish your areas of strength and weakness to optimize your processes while maintaining full alignment with your overall business strategy.

Exhibit 6.1 RCI Analysis

	Reactive	Preventive	Optimize
Obtain and Assess Data	What is happening now in our organization?	What can we prevent from happening?	How can we get to where we want to be?
Evaluate Opportunities	What does the data tell us is causing issues?	Where do we have opportunities to negate those issues?	Where do we have opportunities to streamline processes?

As administrators, directors, and managers, we are looking to ensure the veracity of the revenue cycle. This can only be achieved through continuous analysis. This section will discuss how to create and maintain a financial BCDR (business continuity and disaster recovery) document, methods to evaluate revenue cycle integrity, and how to use technology to automate the alerting of financial warning signs.

6.1 The Financial BCDR

A BCDR document is a "what if" preparation guide for your organization. Most BCDRs will include step-by-step processes to maintain business continuity or recover from a large disaster from a physical operations and HIPAA-compliant standpoint. This can include preparations for everything from facilities damaged by tornadoes to electrical downtime or power surges. BCDRs are designed to ensure intentionality in actions and behaviors in a moment of crisis or immediately following, and to do so, they are created well in advance. For example, the CDC has a protocol for clinical operations in the event of a zombie apocalypse.[1] A zombie apocalypse may be unlikely, but the CDC's joke drew the attention it sought to this urgent need. We must prepare for all potentialities. The 2020 pandemic lasted far longer than anyone thought it would and its ripples extended to healthcare facilities all over the world. We learned much during this time, including how to pivot to work-from-home and how to keep patients and staff safe. We also learned that many of us were not financially ready for a cash flow interruption of this scale and nature.

No one had a pandemic in their 2020 roadmap or BCDR. Some, however, did have a plan for what to do if an emergent closure of offices occurred. These facilities quickly pivoted, and in the end their revenue losses were not as significant as others.

In the first 30 days of the pandemic, Avera Health set up its 24-hour COVID hotline, was the first in the state to be verified by the South Dakota Department of Health for COVID testing, and expanded virtual visits so patients could safely see their provider from home. In addition, within the first days of the pandemic, Avera's information technology team enabled hundreds of employees to begin working from home.[2] These are the results of preparedness.

In order to create something meaningful, your financial BCDR has to be generic enough to apply to a variety of circumstances while remaining achievable, scalable and realistic.

Financial BCDR Areas

Your FBCDR should include, at minimum, how your facility will function in the following unpredictable circumstances:

1. Immediate loss of provider (full-time or part-time)
2. Closure of a single location
3. Closure of the entire facility
4. Unanticipated closure of a critical business associate
5. Critical failure of a mechanical, electrical, or plumbing system
6. Downtime of essential equipment (computer, testing machines, radiology equipment, etc.)
7. Early replacement of large or costly items
8. Large malpractice case judgment
9. Ransomware attack
10. HIPAA breach and associated fines
11. Other large regulatory requirements or fines
12. Sudden double-digit increase in:
    a. Patients seen
    b. Supply costs (medical or administrative)
    c. Base rent costs

Next, you should define what "function" realistically means for each of these areas and potential events as well as the minimum, likely, and maximum financial impact to the organization. Your end goal is to outline the steps toward financial stability as quickly as possible so you don't lose pennies in the pivot.

Example:

Adverse Event: Immediate Loss of a Provider.

Details: A long-term, full-time provider unexpectedly dies, leaving behind thousands of patients who now need to transition to another primary care provider.

<u>Functional</u>: In this type of adverse event, "functional" means we are able to transition 100% of patients to a provider at the same or similar level of care within our facility.

<u>Steps:</u>

1. Reduced attrition:
   a. Staff has a clear understanding of what to say to patients who call with questions
   b. Notification has been submitted to all patients through multiple methods (phone/portal/website/etc.)
2. Reduce financial disruption:
   a. Identify outstanding claims for submission
   b. Expand hours temporarily to accommodate patient reschedules
   c. Achieve stability during recruiting at minimum expense (i.e., avoid high-cost locum tenens or temp staff where possible)
3. Minimize risk:
   a. Ensure operations team immediately processes termination of provider access and collects any facility-granted devices which may grant PHI access
   b. Obtain and destroy any remaining business cards, prescription pads, or other materials that would allow someone to impersonate the provider if these items were merely disposed in the trash
   c. Inform payers, licensing boards, insurance carriers and specialty associations so accounts can be closed accordingly
   d. Use technology to:
      i. Prevent selection of provider in upcoming appointments that may be listed recurrently
      ii. Prevent advanced practice clinicians (APCs) from selecting this provider as an "incident-to" billing option

Exhibit 6.2 FBCDR Example

Adverse Event	Example	Define Functional	Minimum Impact	Likely Impact	Maximum Impact
Immediate loss of provider (full-time or part-time)	Long-term FT provider dies unexpectedly	Able to see all new and existing patients within two weeks	Longer patient wait times and associated patient frustration	Some attrition of new patients and opportunity cost	Loss of existing and new patients including associated revenue

Steps for Achievement: To be able to see all existing and new patients within two weeks of original or prospective DOS, office will immediately need to extend office hours and potentially open temporary weekend hours until a replacement can be found. **Project Lead:** Practice Administrator

1. Evaluate current hours and expand where able
2. Discuss temporary hours and need to employees and providers
3. Develop approved patient communications to distribute in writing and via electronic means (hold music messages, patient portal, text, etc.) for patient communication
4. Contact current patients on schedule to reschedule
   a. Have staff prepared with how to respond if the patient wants to transfer care and how they can contact the former provider
5. Update website to further public transparency
6. Notify licensing bodies of employment separation or death
7. Notify payers/networks

The above table is an example of how you can document the steps required to take action in the event of an unpredictable situation. Of course, the internal documents you prepare can be more detailed – for example, you may be able to dig into the communication templates or contact information for payers/networks. The format may vary – perhaps it is a Word document or a SharePoint file. What matters most is that the information is accurate, usable, and available to staff in the event of this type of situation. In addition, it is very important to note who should be responsible for taking the lead on these tasks. That person should have the:

1) Authority to implement the changes needed

2) Ability to delegate where required

3) Accountability of documentation and follow-up

4) Responsibility to structure a plan back to normal state

The circumstances documented in your FBCDR may not ever occur. If they do, however, this document will save you significant time and administrative burden in deciding next steps.

6.2 A New Perspective on A/R Evaluation

Improving A/R evaluation in part means recognizing that the world today is much different than it was when the 30-day A/R buckets were first structured. Most organizations prioritize A/R based on the date of service or the total charges. The challenge with evaluating by either of these methods is that neither truly relays the value of the claims being worked. To truly prioritize A/R management in the way that is most beneficial for your practice, we first need to shake up the traditional A/R buckets, then we need to tackle the methodology of our prioritization processes.

New A/R Buckets

The traditional buckets for A/R are used so widely that most of us know them without referring to our reports:

- 0 – 30 days
- 31 – 60 days
- 61 – 90 days
- 91 – 120 days
- 120+ days

For decades, bucketing our accounts receivable in these date ranges worked well to grant insight into the velocity of our revenue cycle. It is now time, though, to shake up our perspective on these buckets. The world has changed since these became a staple. We are no longer waiting for the post office to deliver our claims to the payer and for the payer's claims to be delivered by the post office back to us. Now, we are submitting claims electronically with real-time payer acceptance and we are receiving responses, sometimes as soon as the same week. So why are we still waiting so long to review A/R?

Within the first traditional A/R bucket (0-30 days), it is entirely reasonable in today's timeline for a claim to have been submitted, adjudicated and submitted to a secondary payer and adjudicated.

Change your perspective on your A/R buckets to consider the following as your new standard:

Exhibit 6.3 Recommended A/R Buckets by Taya & Kem

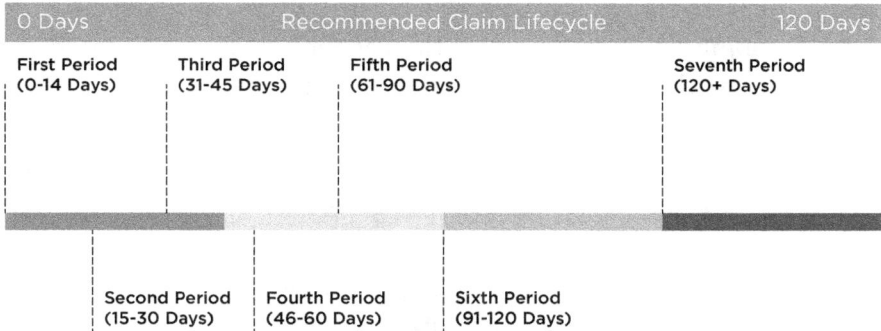

0 Days	Recommended Claim Lifecycle	120 Days

First Period (0-14 Days)	Third Period (31-45 Days)	Fifth Period (61-90 Days)	Seventh Period (120+ Days)

Second Period (15-30 Days)	Fourth Period (46-60 Days)	Sixth Period (91-120 Days)

Activities by Period

- First Period – In this timeframe the claim should be submitted to the primary payer and initial responses may already be coming in.
- Second Period – In the second timeframe, preliminary adjudications should be in, which opens the opportunity to submit to the next area of responsibility (secondary payer, patient, etc.). This is also the first opportunity to begin appealing denied claims.
- Third Period – In this timeframe, adjudications from secondary payers should begin arriving, which means the practice can begin billing for patient responsibilities unless a tertiary insurance needs to be billed.
- Fourth Period – Most payers will have submitted their adjudication by this point. If not, this is a good point for staff to begin outreach.
- Fifth, Sixth, and Seventh Periods – These align with the traditional set of A/R periods.

The sooner you review adjudicated claims, the sooner you can appeal where necessary or bill the patient where needed. Consider the following scenario:

Scenario:

A patient comes in and gives their insurance information. It is checked through the eligibility and benefits verification system and found to be current on that date of service. The patient is seen and the claim is submitted. Five days later the patient's insurance retroactively terminates and the patient's claim is denied as a non-covered service.

Challenges:

Under the traditional bucket review process, your practice could potentially see this patient again before realizing the issue. Even if the issue is realized before the next visit, if you haven't identified the unpaid charges, you've missed an opportunity to collect the patient's responsibility for the first visit when they arrive for their next visit.

The sooner you are able to take action on the adjudication, the stronger your revenue cycle model will be.

Prioritizing A/R

High-value claims are important because they represent the biggest return on your collection efforts. So how do we define "high value"? In order to understand the value of your claims, you need to determine two amounts: the cost of working denials and the worth of the claim. The first can be a bit challenging to identify. Basically, you need to identify what it costs to work claims at various stages: 1st appeal, 2nd appeal, etc., because this will inform when claims should no longer be chased. In addition, identify what your average loaded cost is to work a denial. This will inform when claims are not worth your effort or should be outsourced.

Next, identify the worth of your claims equated to the allowable amount. What can we potentially receive if we achieve collections success? You should be able to find your allowable amounts in your payer contracts. If you cannot locate them, contact the payer for a copy of your fee schedule. Once you have your loaded costs as well as the claim worth, you can determine the value of each claim.

Exhibit 6.4 Hypothetical Prioritization Chart

Procedure	Avg Cost to work	Allowable	Value	Priority
CPT 1	50.00	75.00	25.00	Low
CPT 2	50.00	195.00	145.00	High
CPT 3	50.00	48.00	–2.00	Outsource

The above table doesn't contain real numbers for cost or allowable amounts, but it does provide a visual into how you can use that information to set priorities for your claims. You can even build the prioritization levels into your reports. Once you know the numbers, you can determine which claims should be worked first, which should be worked second, and which should potentially be outsourced to lower-cost service providers where possible.

When we look at our A/R sooner and prioritize the work with strategy, we help to stabilize the revenue cycle model while ensuring that we are acting as quickly as possible on the areas that have the most value to the organization.

6.3 Dealing with Bad Debt

"Bad debt" is the go-to industry term for patient A/R that is past due. Define standard internal criteria for when accounts should be considered bad debt and what next actions should be taken. Most organizations outsource their bad debt collections to a collection agency.

If outsourcing, make sure to establish criteria that define success for your organization. For example, establish thresholds between payment plan and write-off, set the terms by which bad debt should be escalated to a legal case, and provide parameters of discounts for the agency to negotiate within. The agency will define what demographic or financial data is needed to transfer an account, but the practice should define the consequences of non-payment.

Keep in mind that once an account has been sent to collections, a contingency fee on any payments made thereafter would apply, even if the patient pays the practice directly.

Agency Assessment

Selecting a collection agency can be challenging. It's important to remember that what you're looking for is an agency who will become a partner in your revenue collection process. In addition to researching capabilities, past performance, and tactics, you will want to review the culture of the organization. Do they align with the community that you support? Do they align to your visions of collection? Will they be aggressive enough in collecting your money? Will they be too aggressive? These are just some of the questions you will want to ask your prospective vendors.

It's not all about the relationship. You don't want an agency that is great on the phone with you but horrible at collecting your money. Look at specific KPIs and practices that you can assess across all the vendors you evaluate. Some KPIs include:[3]

- Recovery Rate
- Time to Collect
- Services Offered
- Fees
- Location
- Tactics
- Method of Upload
- Method and Frequency of Reporting
- Methods of Payment
- Credit Reporting
- Contract Terms

Formulas

You should review the performance of your collection agency annually at minimum. When evaluating, do not rely solely upon the metrics they provide. Do your own analysis to confirm. Here are three commonly used formulas to use in your analysis:[4]

Gross Collections Formula = Total Collected ÷ Total Debt Sent for Collections

This is a quick and dirty analysis: what did we send you to get and what of that did you get?

Net Cost of Collection Formula = Total Collected − Fees ÷ Total Debt Sent for Collections

This is a net profit analysis against your debt collections program. Are you paying more to collect your money than you are receiving? Is there a large-enough margin that there aren't concerns going forward?

Net Collections Formula = Total Collected ÷ Total Collectible Sent for Collections

This is a bit more complex. What did we send you to collect? What of that was collectable? What portion of what was collectable did you get? For example, if a patient files for bankruptcy collection proceedings, collections attempts should cease in order to follow the bankruptcy proceedings instead. In these situations, the collections agency is not at fault because that debt is uncollectable.

If you perform your due diligence up front and regularly communicate with and evaluate your collections agency, you can build a long-term relationship. If you do build a long-term relationship, then make sure that you compare your annual findings across the previous 3-5 years. If you notice a trend in decreased performance, then you may need to reevaluate your relationship.

Critical Steps for Bad-Debt Management

The most pivotal steps for bad-debt management are:

1. Early identification: the sooner you identify rising patient costs the better you will be able to prevent large balances from accruing

2. Effective collection: educate internal staff and bad debt agencies on what is expected and what is acceptable for collecting past due balances in alignment with your organization's mission, vision, and values

3. Regulatory and legislative compliance: ensure adherence to fair debt collections practices, bankruptcy laws, and other regulations that require specific management processes for bad debt collection

4. Optimized use of technology: implement alerts in your practice management system for rising bad debt costs, automate messages to patients that offer payment plans, and set up automatic patient payments

5. Communicate costs to patients early: when patients know the cost of the care, they are more likely to pay for their care and less likely to unnecessarily utilize costly services, items or procedures

The best method for preventive bad-debt management is:

1. Price transparency: communicating what patients may be responsible for clearly and in writing has proven to increase their understanding and likelihood of payment

2. Financial hardship programs: these have methods by which you can validate when patients have true financial disparity early on before large balances are accrued

3. Pre-defined payment plans: if patients need to individually speak with the billing manager to set up payment plans, this misses an opportunity for other staff members to get patients set up on payment plans. For example, if a patient is at the front desk and reminded of a balance due, setting up a payment plan at the point of care speeds up the time to A/R capture.

6.4 Applying Revenue Integrity Metrics Across the Full RCM Cycle

In order to apply organizational metrics that help strengthen the revenue cycle, you have to formulate a strategy that considers every step.

That means looking at every function and creating a metric that drives toward operational improvement and increased revenue cycle integrity. Revenue Integrity (RI) is a critical component of the revenue cycle and financial management of any healthcare organization. A successful RI program will identify not only sources of leakage but the root cause of those sources. It will then apply internal controls that may be replicated across workstreams. The integrity component of an RI program includes predicting future trends and external changes that may impact internal controls and either adjust or evolve to new needs. A few drivers that will affect an RI program include cyber-security threats, workforce changes, transition of Electronic Health Records (EHR) and/or practice management (PM) software, regulatory compliance changes, technology service innovations, payer reimbursement guideline adjustments and patient care trends.

If your organization does not have a formal RI program, there are most likely processes in place that are based on ethical business standards to ensure compliance, efficiencies in workflows and operations as well as optimizing income potential. As you begin to develop your formal revenue integrity (RI) program, consider:

1. Ethical business standards, policies and processes that keep your organization compliant with regulatory agencies' requirements as well as insurance reimbursement guidelines.

2. Develop and continuously re-engineer internal operations to adapt to internal workforce/providers and external patient/customer needs that streamline workflows to allow for duplication and automation of processes.

3. Optimize earning potential by following reimbursement guidelines, implementing service enhancers, capturing all billable services and optimizing technology.

Most healthcare organizations are familiar with the "revenue generating balancing act" – counting dollars without crossing the line and breaking the rules. We must always deploy ethical decision-making when using healthcare services as a revenue generator. Internally auditing your organization's financial business practices is essential to ensuring that compliance and ethical standards are applied company-wide. Instituting a culture of compliance is a key factor within a Revenue Integrity (RI) program. Take a look at the below Revenue Integrity wheel.

Exhibit 6.5 Revenue Integrity Wheel

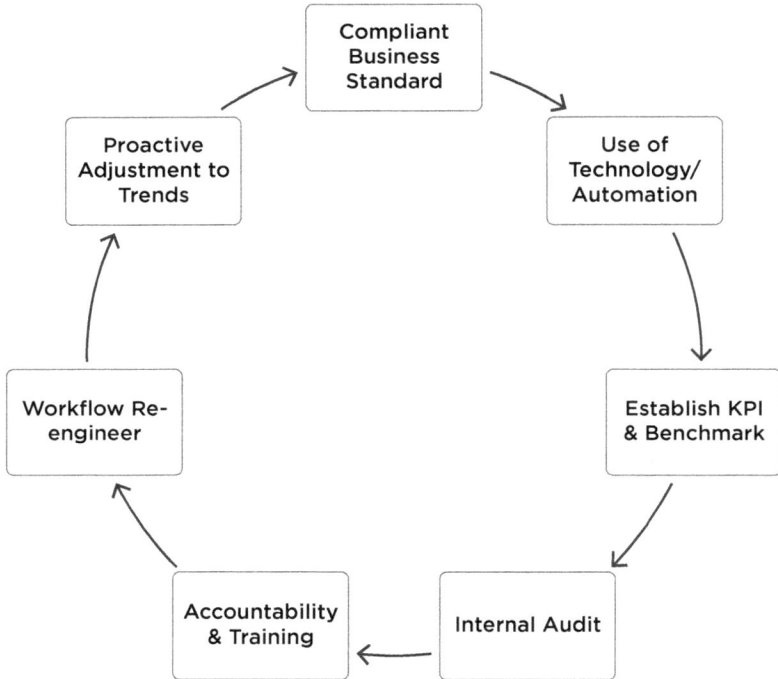

Revenue Integrity Application

Let's apply Revenue Integrity (RI) principles to a financial scenario.

A large multi-specialty practice cannot put their finger on why their inpatient monthly financial projections do not meet expectations. After an internal review, it has been found that there has not been a significant change in unique visits or a decrease in the number of providers rendering services. The billing department has complained that they need more staff to assist with data entry for inpatient hospital services. The current inpatient billing process calls for physicians to drop off daily superbills to the charge entry staff, who are responsible for using shared access to the hospital's EHR to gather demographic face sheets for each patient's encounter. The face sheet is then given to staff members to register patients into the practice's EHR. There are assigned charge entry staff to enter, scrub and submit claims. Ultimately, there are several opportunities within the organization's workflows to deploy RI protocols.

- Compliant Business Standard
    - Current – Hospital charges will be billed within 48 hours of receipt of face sheets
    - RI Application – Hospital charges are 30% of practice revenue and require a hybrid manual and automated process for data collection, validation, entry, reconciliation and submission that includes input and monitoring between physicians, billing staff and leadership

- Use of Technology/ Automation
    - Current – Manual process of hospital superbills given to staff from physicians for manual data entry
    - RI Application – Create staff role-specific hospital EMR/PM software access for visit data gathering. Create a matrix of data elements needed from the hospital's system for billing. Audit staff access quarterly to remove expired access.

- Establish KPI & Benchmark
    - Current – Director of Finance projects the number of unique hospital visits using the physician call schedule.
    - RI Application – Create hospital visit benchmark using the last 12-24 months of unique encounters. Implement key performance indicators (KPI) to track performance and to re-establish new benchmarks as needed.

- Internal Audit
  - Current – Staff run hospital billing productivity reports by provider.
  - RI Application – Create a reconciliation report to internally audit encounters against billed services. Assess hospital billing process, document findings, and identify best practices.
- Accountability & Training
  - Current – Not in place.
  - RI Application – Utilize best practices from internal audit to create policy documents and procedure documents for each step of the hospital billing process to include provider documentation. Assign staff to necessary steps. Create and deploy training program. Update job descriptions. Create a lookback period.
- Workflow Re-engineer
  - Current – Disjointed manual processes.
  - RI Application – Utilize updated policy documents and training to include automation within the new workflow. Request staff feedback on new processes for adjustments as needed.
- Proactive Adjustment to Trends
  - Current – Not in place.
  - RI Application – Utilize workflow assessment to identify workstreams that will be impacted by changes in regulations, software access, staffing changes, and service delivery. Create flexible policy and procedures for these areas.

Evaluating for Integrity

Focus on areas where your metrics, KPIs, and dashboards indicate opportunities for improvement, and perform an analysis that identifies your reactive, preventive, and optimization approaches.

Evaluation happens in three phases:

1. Reactive

2. Preventive

3. Optimize

We need to look at each phase through two primary activities **obtaining/assessing data** and **evaluating opportunities**.

Exhibit 6.6 Reactive, Preventive, and Optimize chart

	Reactive	Preventive	Optimize
Obtain and Assess Data	What is happening now in our organization?	What can we prevent from happening?	How can we get to where we want to be?
Evaluate Opportunities	What does the data tell us is causing issues?	Where do we have opportunities to negate those issues?	Where do we have opportunities to streamline processes?

Reactive Phase

In this section we want to identify what is currently happening in our organization and what that data tells us. This is the stabilization phase. Investigating data often identifies areas where immediate action needs to be taken. That quick reaction should focus on stopping the bleeding. Think of this section like an emergency response.

Preventive Phase

In this phase, we are looking at preventing these situations from happening again. So, we want to look at the data and determine the root cause. Determine what can be prevented and evaluate the opportunities to negate those issues.

Optimize Phase

This is the fun section. This is where we evaluate our data a third time. We have stabilized any issues and are preventing what we can. Now it's time to determine what is considered "optimal" for the given focus area. Once optimal has been defined, determine how to get to optimal and the processes that can be streamlined to create opportunities to achieve optimal status.

Exhibit 6.7 A/R Evaluation for Revenue Cycle Integrity

	Reactive	Preventive	Optimize
Obtain and Assess Data	What are our current A/R balances? How are we grouping our A/R buckets? Is this sufficient for what we need to evaluate?	Of the A/R buckets we've evaluated, how often are we able to recoup the claims with 90+ days in A/R? What are the issues presented by those claims?	What do we consider "optimal" for A/R balances by bucket? Where can we integrate points to inject processes to reach optimal?
Evaluate Opportunities	What can we infer from this data? What does it tell us about our current processes within the revenue cycle model?	Where do we have opportunities to prevent/negate the issues we are seeing? What processes can we implement to support these efforts?	Minimize redundancy in processes/workflows while optimizing accuracy wherever possible.

In the above example, questions have been included to indicate how you should approach each phase. Remember to obtain and assess data, evaluate opportunities, and effect change for each phase before moving on to the next. In each phase, the reevaluation of data is critical because it serves as a lookback point to ensure that you are progressing toward your goals.

As you evaluate the data, consider KPIs that can support your decision-making processes across the financial continuum:

- Unique Patient Visits – help to identify staffing needs, room utilization, appointment optimization
- Diagnosis Utilization – helps identify which high-risk patients are most prevalent in the community
- Referring Provider – identifies patient sourcing and potential collaboration opportunities
- Adjustments – indicates collections performance, opportunity to enhance the specificity of adjustment codes
- Payer Mix & Payer Income – grants guidance on participation needs and opportunities for fee schedule negotiations
- Patient Age & Gender – can support preventive services marketing efforts and community outreach, aids identification of supply/equipment needs

These are examples of just a handful of areas that you should evaluate to strengthen the overall integrity of your revenue cycle. Evaluate against industry benchmarks as well as your own benchmarks for past performance.

Benchmarking

Quick reminder on benchmarks: a "percentile" reflects where a score stands relative to other scores. So, for example, the 95th percentile means your score is greater than 95% of the other scores.

To calculate percentiles, use the formula $\mathbf{n = (P \div 100)\ x\ N}$ where 'n' = the ranking of a given value (smallest to largest), 'P' = the percentile, and 'N' = the number of values in the data set. For more information on percentiles, refer back to section 3.7.

Exhibit 6.8 Mean/Average (Repeat)

Mean	Average
Standard Deviation	Distance of values from the Mean
25th Percentile	Low
50th Percentile	Median / Middle
90th Percentile	High

Prior to leveraging benchmark data, it's important that you:

1. Define your metrics

2. Identify available data

3. Select the timeframe

4. Create your internal goal

5. Identify who you will measure against

   a. Look at credible resources like MGMA's DataDive, CMS' Data Warehouse, or AAPC's data

   b. Look at your specialty association data

   c. Look for facilities that are similar (like sized, like services, similar geographic regions, etc.)

After you've done these things, you can begin to compare your performance.

6.5 Using Technology to Automate the Alerting of Financial Warning Signs

Whether technology will be a liability or an asset will all come down to utilization, training, and your alerting methodology. When we think of the alerting process in technology, especially in health care, we tend to think of the alerts that pop up in the electronic health record system. It's no secret that so many of these have led to alert fatigue for providers as well as staff due to overuse. For that reason alone, it is exceedingly important to make sure that the alerts being created are functioning in a useful, timely, minimalistic way. Some things can and should be automated whereas others should not or cannot; success occurs in the balance between those.

When you're deciding what should be an alert versus what is something that you should just report on, think in terms of traffic signals. There are some circumstances in which you're just going to have normal rules to follow and these are items that you should be reporting on in your dashboard – for example, if you have patients who have Medicaid, that doesn't require an alert. There is a section in the practice management system to document and review the patient's insurance/funding source. Where there are already fields in existence that should be utilized, think of those as traffic lights. It is the responsibility of the person using the road to look at the traffic lights and assess how that impacts the next step.

An alert, on the other hand, should be thought of like an ambulance siren indicating that you need to pull over to the shoulder because a unique or more complex situation is occurring. An alert is most helpful when it's based on a series of rules and not just one. For example, if you have a patient with a high balance whose insurance has just terminated and employment is listed as 'null', perhaps an alert should indicate that financial hardship discussions may need to be had. Another example of a good financial alert is if you have a very complicated case that is being managed through one employee primarily; this can indicate to staff not to waste their time trying to read back through the communications and instead to transfer that call to the most accurate person. When we think of financial alerts, we want to make sure we are not mixing up custom alerts with those that provide basic information. Basic information alerts are typically those that are canned within the practice management system already. Using alerts to train staff in proper chart review or account review is not ideal. Instead, we should focus on processes and opportunities for staff education. This is how we separate between alert fatigue and a successful alerting program.

Financial Trend Alerts

Developing alerts for financial trends can also be very helpful. If you have created a set of dashboards or reports that you look at with a given frequency, that provides you the information required to run the practice day-to-day and also to identify potential future financial impact. When we look at financial trend alerting, we want the system to identify more information than we can quickly identify ourselves. For example, if we are reviewing days in A/R, we don't want an alert to simply tell us what the days in A/R for >90 days are. We can easily see that ourselves in our reports and dashboards. Here are some examples of more useful A/R alerts which can be implemented:

- If days in A/R for Payer exceed sixty days and no 835 has been received, send notification to billing manager
- If the number of days between date of service and date of claims submission exceeds seven days, send alert to billing manager
- If more than two claims were retroactively denied by the same payer for the same procedure code, send alert to practice manager
- If first pass claims payment rate drops below 85%, send alert to billing manager

In each of these examples, alerts for very specific situations are created to help notify leadership of trends that it would take them longer to identify on their own.

Beyond the Concept

As you modify or develop an internal revenue integrity program, take into consideration all the aspects discussed in this chapter, especially as it relates to the overall Revenue Cycle Model. Each component of the revenue cycle will impact an organization's financial success. Incorporating Revenue Integrity protocols into your Revenue Cycle promotes an "Identify, Fix and Look-back" model for ensuring issues do not persist. The below RI standards may be used within an internal RI program.

Exhibit 6.9 Revenue Integrity Standards

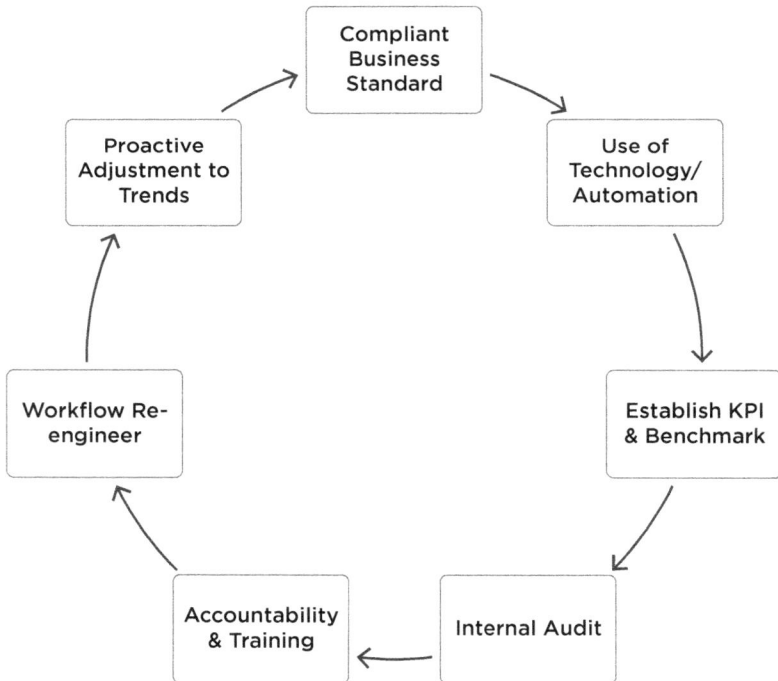

Revenue Integrity Standards

1. Create business standards that are ethical and based on regulations that if competing or overlapping with other– such as state and federal guidelines–are clearly explained with a business goal, purpose and expectation.

2. Optimize technology in all areas that could be automated to focus human capital for decision-making rather than checking off boxes and clicking through screens. Automation promotes error reduction and faster workflows.

3. Establishing Key Performance Indicators and Benchmarks ensures that your organization is aware of its goals – awareness precedes success.

4. Routine audits for coding, collections, payer receipts, compliance, and key internal processes identify inefficiencies, non-compliance, and areas that require improvement.

5. Training programs may be customized by using audit results. Since the findings are specific to your organization, they also allow for development of revised expectations by workforce members and providers. In order to hold individuals accountable for performance, standards must be communicated and training on best practices should be available.

6. Re-engineering workflows is not for the weak. You must be all-in and completely knowledgeable of the pros and cons of impending changes. All stakeholders involved in a workflow should be consulted and buy-in obtained so that everyone "owns" the workflow.

7. At its core, Revenue Integrity is a proactive approach to avoid revenue leakage. Rather than waiting for non-payment to occur, we implement processes to ensure revenue is not impacted again in the future. In order to make adjustments to trends that could bring in new revenue for your organization, one must be on the hunt for new information, and bring it back to stakeholders.

Curating Alerts

Curating the alerts for your practice management system will not be a one and done activity. This is an area that requires look-backs and review to ensure continuous optimization. To set up meaningful financial alerts, you will need to:[5]

1) **Include the appropriate stakeholders.** You will definitely need leadership present but there is often value in including the staff members who actually work claims as well.

2) **Evaluate what already exists.** It is likely that you've already implemented some financial alerts in your system. Do not fall into the "this is the way we've always done it" trap. Critically review each alert that exists and verify if they are useful. Are they all truly important sirens alerting you to complex situations? Or are some of them merely acting as a stop-gap for substandard staff training or inefficient processes?

3) **Perform a technology review.** What is your system capable of doing? Even if you've had the system for a long time, chances are there have been updates. Are you using the system to the fullest extent of its capabilities? What are the limitations on setting up alerts? What is the process? Does it require additional cost? Can you create the rules for the alerts on your own?

4) **Assess what you need.** Again, not everything needs to be an alert. So, what is going to be most useful for your team in order to progress toward your strategic revenue cycle goals? Look at your grouped denials and long-standing A/R claims and ask what alerts could have driven quicker remediation?

5) **Look-back.** After you change your alerts, you will find that some are helpful, some are not, and some are flat out annoying. Adjust these as needed but make sure that the period of time the alert was implemented isn't too short to have truly informed you sufficiently.

6.7 Case Study

Background:

A specialty health system contracted with an outsourced consulting firm to identify and resolve revenue integrity pitfalls as well as to collect on unpaid claims. The outsourced collections resolution team initiated clean-up by working 150+ aging A/R to identify collectible and uncollectible monies as well as to identify and resolve unworked denial trends. The team began noticing certain claims had not been submitted, even though there was proof that the batches were submitted.

Investigation:

The unpaid claims were being tracked to Payer EDI #60032. A report was run for this specific payer for all dates of service. It was determined that no claims were submitted to this payer. Upon investigation of the system settings for this payer, a claims hold was set to [YES]. The system settings for payers had not been reviewed since inception several years prior. During the investigation, it was identified that there were duplicates of the same payer with varying claims addresses and EDI numbers. The final investigation resulted in a thorough audit of all payer profile settings for accuracy and compilation of duplicates.

Outcome:

The system setting profile for the original payer that was not receiving claims was corrected, address updated, credentialing and provider enrollment confirmed, and EDI # confirmed. Claims hold was reset to [NO]. Claims hold setting for all payers was reviewed and default was set to [NO]. Claims on hold were scrubbed and submitted based on timely filing guidelines. A revenue integrity protocol was instituted to ensure that payer profile settings are audited twice a year, access to make payer profile changes was limited to department leadership (as it was discovered that all staff had these permissions previously), and protocols were developed and communicated to staff on how to address non-payments of this type in the future.

Notes

1. CDC. https://emergency.cdc.gov/cerc/cerccorner/article_050918.asp
2. Avera. https://www.avera.org/news-media/news/2022/second-anniversary-of-covid. Accessed on 1.18.23.
3. Tolliver K and Moheiser T. Revenue Cycle Management: Don't Get Lost in the Financial Maze. MGMA. p. 257-258.

4. Tolliver K, Gordon T. Revenue Cycle Management: Don't Get Lost in the Financial Maze. p. 260.
5. Medical Economics. https://www.medicaleconomics.com/view/making-ehr-alerts-work-your-practice

Index

Page numbers in **bold** are for the exhibits and figures references.

Centers for Medicare and Medicaid Services (or CMS), 16-17, 20, 45, 50, 52, 78, 95, 110, 116, 154

Certified coder (also known as certified professional coder, CPC), 26-27

Charge entry, **53**, 191

Charity Care, 102, 104, 106, **159**

Chart, 140, **141**, 171, **185**, **193**, 197

Check-in / Check-out, **53**, 103, 122, 127, 170, 173-174

Chronic Care Management, 110, 120, 127

Claim
    claims billing, **4**
    claims payment, 66, 77, 197
    claims processing, **19**, **64**, 101, 135
    claims submission, **63**, 177, 197

Clearinghouse, **63**, **76**, 78, 144, 150

Clinical
    Clinical Decision Support, 50, **116**
    Clinical Quality Measure (CQM), 47, 51-52
    Clinically Integrated Network (CIN), 50, 52, 68

CMS (Centers for Medicare and Medicaid Services), 16, 47, 50, 95, 116, **116**, 122, 125, 154, 171. *See also* Medicare; Medicaid

Code or Coding, **19**, 25, 58, 67, 71, 76, 78, 87-88, 111, **116**, 123, **125-126**, 127, **128**, 135, 159, **159**, 199

Coinsurance, **4**, 48, 65, 99

Collections, 165, 167, 170, 185-186, 194, 201

Compliance, 75, 82-83, 86, 88-89, **129**, 141, 145, 153. *See also* Risk or Risk Management

Consumer, 28, 48, 62, 86, 117, **121**, 168. *See also* Consumer-driven

Consumer-driven, 48

Contract (or contracts)
    breach of contract, 172
    contract evaluation, contract language, 14, 55-56, 58-59, 62, **62**, 64, 67, 170

contract terms, 13, 58, 62, 66, 186
    payer contracting, 56, 66
    payer contracts, 59, 76, 172, 184
    risk-based contracts, 21, 23, 112-113

Copayment, 99, 104, **121**, 171

CPT, **19**, 57, **64**, 67, 71, **81**, 83, **111**, 115, **116**, **125-126**, 128, 135, **185**

Credentialing, 76, 88, 201

Credit, 35, 140, 166, 186
    credit card, 48, **75**, 78, **81**, 129, 131, 167, 169

D

Dashboard(s), **53**, 133, **134**, 135-136, 142, 192, 196-197

Debt
    bad debt, 185, 187
    debt collection, 159, 166, 187-188
    debt collector, 166
    total debt, 186

Deductibles, 35, 37, 104, 171-172

Denials, **4**, 45, 83, 101, 135, 150, 200

Department of Health and Human Services, 49, 88-89

Deposit, 131

Diagnosis, **19**, 25, 123, 194

Documentation, 26, 123, 125-126, 128, 161, 181, 192

Durable Medical Equipment (DME), **17**, 99

E

EFT (electronic funds transfer), 59, 77, 79, 130

EHR, EMR, Electronic Health Record, Electronic Medical Record, 47, 50, 52, **69**, 96, 101, 116-117, **116**, 128, 142, 189, 191

Eligibility, **4**, **53**, 92, 104, 159, 184

Employer, 28, 58, 66, 129

Evaluation and Management (E&M), 58, 67, 111, 128

www.ingramcontent.com/pod-product-compliance
Lightning Source LLC
Chambersburg PA
CBHW060554220326
41598CB00024B/3097